INTRODUCTION

I magine waking up one day to find that your legs have become heavy, swollen, and painful, making it a struggle to move freely. Or imagine feeling like your arms are encased in an invisible weight, making simple tasks like lifting a glass of water seem like an impossible feat. For many individuals, this isn't a mere exercise of imagination; it's their daily reality.

Lipedema and lymphedema are two relentless conditions that silently affect the lives of millions. These conditions, while distinct in their origins, share a common thread— swelling. Swelling disrupts lives, burdens the body, and challenges the spirit.

Lipedema, often misdiagnosed and misunderstood, hides beneath the surface, where an abnormal accumulation of fat cells in the legs and sometimes the arms leads to aching limbs and an overwhelming sense of frustration. It predominantly targets women, often making its debut during life-altering moments like puberty, pregnancy, or menopause.

On the other hand, lymphedema, with its unyielding accumulation of lymphatic fluid, casts a shadow on one or more limbs or even other unsuspecting parts of the body. The consequences are relentless—swollen limbs, compromised mobility, and increased vulnerability to infections.

The journey of those afflicted by these conditions is one of resilience and hope, but it's also a path laden with unanswered questions. In the pursuit of solutions, many turn to conventional medicine, rehabilitation therapies, or surgical interventions, yet one crucial element often remains overlooked—the transformative power of nutrition.

In this comprehensive guide, we embark on a journey of discovery, exploring the profound impact of nutrition on lymphedema and lipedema management. We'll delve into the intricate workings of the lymphatic system, decode the mysteries of inflammation, and uncover the dietary strategies that can make a world of difference.

The pages that follow will not only provide you with a roadmap to alleviate the challenges of lymphedema and lipedema but will also empower you with knowledge, practical advice, and inspiration. Whether you are personally navigating these conditions or seeking to support a loved one, this book is your beacon of hope in the journey towards better health and a brighter future.

Join us as we embark on a transformative exploration of the Lymphedema and Lipedema Nutrition Guide—a journey towards relief, resilience, and renewal.

CHAPTER 1:

*Understanding Lymphedema
and Lipedema*

What Is Lipedema?

Lipedema is a chronic and often misunderstood medical condition characterised by the abnormal accumulation of fat cells, primarily in the legs and sometimes in the arms. It predominantly affects women and can have a profound impact on physical and emotional well-being.

Causes of lipedema

Several factors may contribute to the development of lipedema, including:

1. Genetics: There is strong evidence to suggest that genetics play a significant role in the development of lipedema. It often runs in families, and individuals with a family history of lipedema are at a higher risk of developing the condition themselves. Specific genetic markers associated with lipedema are still being studied.

2. Hormonal Factors: Hormonal fluctuations, particularly those associated with puberty, pregnancy, and menopause, seem to trigger or exacerbate lipedema symptoms in

many cases. The condition predominantly affects women, suggesting a hormonal influence.

3. Hormone Receptors: Some researchers have proposed that lipedema may be related to hormonal receptors in adipose tissue (fat cells). These receptors could make fat cells more susceptible to hormonal changes and the subsequent accumulation of fat.

4. Inflammation: Chronic inflammation may contribute to the development and progression of lipedema. Inflammation can affect blood vessels and lymphatic function, potentially leading to fluid retention and fat deposition in affected areas.

5. Lymphatic Dysfunction: The lymphatic system plays a crucial role in maintaining fluid balance in the body. Some researchers believe that impaired lymphatic function may contribute to the accumulation of fluid and fat in the tissues, although it is not clear if this is a cause or an effect of lipedema.

6.   Other Factors: While less well-established, other factors such as trauma, infections, or metabolic factors have also been suggested as potential contributors to lipedema. These factors may interact with genetic predispositions and hormonal changes.

It's important to note that while these factors are associated with lipedema, the condition's exact cause is likely a combination of genetic, hormonal, and environmental factors. Moreover, not all individuals with these risk factors will develop lipedema, and the condition can vary widely in its severity and progression among affected individuals.

Risk factors for lipedema

Several risk factors have been identified that may increase the likelihood of developing the condition. These risk factors include:

1. Gender: Lipedema overwhelmingly affects women, with estimates suggesting that approximately 11% of women may have some degree of lipedema. While it can occur in men, it is rare. The female predominance suggests that hormonal factors may play a role in the development of lipedema.

2. Family History: There is a strong genetic component to lipedema. Individuals with a family history of lipedema are at a higher risk of developing the condition themselves. This genetic predisposition suggests that specific genetic factors may contribute to the risk of lipedema.

3. Hormonal Changes: Lipedema often becomes more pronounced or worsens during significant hormonal changes, such as puberty, pregnancy, and menopause. Hormonal fluctuations may trigger or exacerbate lipedema symptoms.

4. Obesity: While lipedema is not caused by obesity, there is a correlation between lipedema and obesity. Many individuals with lipedema are overweight or obese. Excess body weight can exacerbate lipedema symptoms, and managing weight can be challenging due to the condition's effects on fat distribution.

5. Age: Lipedema typically begins to manifest during or after puberty and may progress over time. It can also become more noticeable with age. However, it is not limited to a specific age group, and cases have been documented in individuals of various ages.

6. Hormonal Disorders: Some individuals with hormonal

disorders, such as polycystic ovary syndrome (PCOS), may be at a higher risk of developing lipedema. Hormonal imbalances associated with these conditions may contribute to fat accumulation.

7. Trauma or Surgery: Some cases of lipedema have been reported following trauma, surgery, or medical procedures. It is thought that physical trauma or surgical interventions may trigger the onset of lipedema in susceptible individuals.

Stages and symptoms

Lipedema is often categorised into different stages based on the severity and progression of the condition. The stages help healthcare professionals assess the extent of the lipedema and plan appropriate treatment strategies. While the staging systems may vary slightly depending on the source, here is a commonly used four-stage classification along with their peculiar symptoms:

Stage 1:

• In the early stage of lipedema, the accumulation of excess fat is relatively mild.

• Symptoms may include a soft, "doughy" feeling to the skin in affected areas.

• Mild tenderness or discomfort may be present but is not usually severe.

• The shape of the limbs may appear relatively normal, with minimal noticeable changes in contour.

Stage 2:

• In this stage, the lipedema fat becomes more pronounced and begins to affect the shape of the limbs.

• There is a noticeable increase in the volume of fat in the legs and sometimes the arms.

• The skin may feel firmer, and there may be areas of nodularity or small, lump-like formations within the fat.

• Tenderness and discomfort become more noticeable, and there may be increased sensitivity to pressure.

• Bruising and easy injury to the affected areas may occur.

Stage 3:

Stage 3 is characterised by a significant increase in the volume of fat and structural changes in the limbs.

• The skin can become more fibrous and may have a "mattress-like" appearance.

• The limbs may appear deformed, with irregular contours and pronounced fatty deposits.

• Pain and discomfort can be moderate to severe, affecting daily activities.

• Mobility and joint problems are more common in this stage.

Stage 4:

• This is the most advanced stage of lipedema, with the most severe fat accumulation and associated symptoms.

• The limbs can be extremely enlarged and misshapen.

• The skin may become thickened and fibrotic, and there may be significant nodularity.

• Severe pain, tenderness, and discomfort are typical, often affecting mobility and quality of life.

• Lymphatic and vascular complications are more likely at this stage.

It's important to note that lipedema does not typically involve the feet, and there is usually a clear demarcation at the ankles. The upper body, including the abdomen and chest, is also typically spared from lipedema fat accumulation.

Diagnosis of lipedema

Diagnosing lipedema typically involves a combination of clinical evaluation, medical history assessment, and, in some cases, imaging studies. Here are the key steps involved in the diagnosis of lipedema:

1. Medical History and Symptom Assessment:

Your healthcare provider will begin by taking a detailed medical history, including any family history of lipedema or related conditions.

They will ask about your symptoms, including when they started, how they have progressed, and any factors that exacerbate or alleviate them.

It's essential to provide information about any medical conditions, surgeries, or traumas that may be relevant to your symptoms.

2. Physical Examination:

A physical examination is a crucial part of the diagnosis. Your healthcare provider will carefully examine the affected areas, such as your legs and sometimes your arms.

They will assess the distribution of fat, looking for characteristic signs of lipedema, including symmetrical fat accumulation, a clear demarcation at the ankles, and the presence of a "doughy" or soft feeling to the skin.

Any tenderness or pain in the affected areas will also be

noted during the examination.

3. Exclusion of Other Conditions:

Lipedema shares some similarities with other conditions, such as lymphedema, obesity, and lipohypertrophy. To confirm a lipedema diagnosis, your healthcare provider will need to rule out these other possibilities.

Imaging studies or additional tests may be conducted to exclude other conditions and provide further evidence of lipedema.

4. Imaging Studies (Optional):

In some cases, imaging studies such as lymphoscintigraphy, MRI (Magnetic Resonance Imaging), or ultrasound may be used to help confirm the diagnosis of lipedema and rule out other conditions.

These imaging tests can provide information about the distribution of fat, the condition of lymphatic vessels, and the absence of other underlying issues.

5. Consultation with a Specialist:

Since lipedema is a relatively rare and often misunderstood condition, it may be beneficial to consult with a specialist experienced in the diagnosis and management of lipedema. These specialists may include dermatologists, vascular surgeons, or lymphatic therapists.

6. Biopsy (Rarely Necessary):

A biopsy of the fat tissue is rarely required for a lipedema diagnosis. However, in some cases, a biopsy may be performed to confirm the diagnosis definitively. This involves taking a small tissue sample from the affected area for laboratory analysis.

Management and treatment of lipedema

The management and treatment of lipedema aim to alleviate symptoms, improve quality of life, and slow down the progression of the condition. Various conservative and surgical approaches can help manage the symptoms and reduce discomfort. The choice of treatment depends on the individual's specific situation and the stage of the condition.

Conservative Management:

Compression Therapy: Wearing graduated compression garments, such as compression stockings or wraps, can help reduce swelling, alleviate discomfort, and improve lymphatic flow. Properly fitted compression garments are essential for effectiveness.

Manual Lymphatic Drainage (MLD) is a specialized massage technique that trained therapists use. It helps stimulate lymphatic flow, reduce fluid buildup, and ease discomfort. MLD is typically part of a comprehensive lipedema management plan.

Exercise: Low-impact exercise, such as swimming, water aerobics, or walking, can improve circulation, promote lymphatic drainage, and support overall health. It's crucial to consult with a healthcare provider or physical therapist to develop an exercise programme tailored to individual capabilities.

Healthy Diet: A balanced diet can help manage weight and reduce inflammation. Focus on whole foods, fruits, vegetables, lean protein, and healthy fats. Avoid excessive sodium intake, as it can contribute to fluid retention.

Lipid-Lowering Medications: In some cases, medications

that help reduce fat levels in the blood, such as statins, may be considered to manage lipedema. This approach is still under investigation.

Surgical Interventions:

Liposuction: Liposuction, specifically water-assisted liposuction (WAL) or tumescent liposuction, can be an effective treatment for advanced stages of lipedema. It involves the removal of excess fat deposits from the affected areas, which can provide significant relief from pain and discomfort. A surgeon with experience in lipedema treatment should perform liposuction.

Psychosocial Support:

Coping with a chronic condition like lipedema can be emotionally challenging. Psychosocial support, such as counselling or support groups, can help individuals manage the emotional aspects of living with lipedema, including body image issues and self-esteem concerns.

Lifestyle Modifications:

Avoiding tight clothing and garments that constrict circulation in the affected areas can help reduce discomfort.

Elevating the legs whenever possible can promote lymphatic drainage and reduce swelling.

Combined Therapies:

A comprehensive approach to lipedema management often combines multiple treatment modalities, including conservative measures, surgery, and lifestyle modifications, tailored to the individual's needs.

Emotional and psychological impact of

lipedema

Lipedema can have a profound emotional and psychological impact on individuals living with the condition. The emotional and psychological challenges often result from a combination of factors, including the physical symptoms, body image concerns, and the chronic nature of the condition.

Body Image Issues:

Lipedema can lead to a distorted body image, as individuals often experience disproportionate fat accumulation in the legs and arms while the upper body remains relatively unaffected.

The visible differences in limb size and shape may lead to feelings of embarrassment, self-consciousness, and negative self-perception.

Low Self-Esteem:

• Individuals with lipedema may develop low self-esteem due to their altered appearance and perceived physical imperfections.

• These feelings of low self-worth can affect relationships, work, and social interactions.

3. Emotional distress:

• Chronic pain, discomfort, and the physical limitations associated with lipedema can lead to emotional distress, including feelings of frustration, sadness, and anger.

Coping with the physical and emotional aspects of the condition can be mentally draining and exhausting.

4. Anxiety and Depression:

• Living with a chronic condition like lipedema can increase the risk of anxiety and depression. The emotional toll of managing the condition, along with the uncertainty of its progression, can contribute to these mental health challenges.

5. Social Isolation:

• Lipedema symptoms may lead to social withdrawal and isolation, as individuals may avoid social situations, exercise, or clothing that highlights their condition.

• Fear of judgement or negative comments from others can further contribute to social isolation.

6. Coping Mechanisms:

• Some individuals may develop maladaptive coping mechanisms, such as emotional eating or avoidance behaviours, as a way to deal with the emotional distress associated with lipedema.

7. Impact on Relationships:

• Lipedema can affect personal relationships, including intimate partnerships, as individuals may struggle with self-confidence and feelings of inadequacy.

• Loved ones may also find it challenging to understand and support those with lipedema.

8. Treatment-Related Stress:

• The pursuit of diagnosis and effective treatment can be stressful and frustrating, as lipedema is often misdiagnosed or poorly understood within the medical community.

It's crucial to address the emotional and psychological aspects of lipedema alongside its physical management. Seeking support from mental health professionals, such as therapists or counsellors, can help individuals cope with emotional challenges and develop healthy strategies for managing stress, anxiety, and depression.

What Is Lymphedema?

Lymphedema is a chronic medical condition characterised by the abnormal accumulation of lymphatic fluid in the tissues, leading to swelling, often in one or more limbs but sometimes affecting other parts of the body as well. This condition occurs when the lymphatic system, a network of vessels and lymph nodes responsible for fluid and immune system function, is compromised or damaged.

Causes of lymphedema

Lymphedema can result from various underlying causes, including:

1. Surgery: Surgical procedures that involve the removal of lymph nodes or damage to the lymphatic vessels can disrupt the normal flow of lymphatic fluid, leading to lymphedema. Common surgeries associated with lymphedema include cancer-related lymph node removal (e.g., mastectomy with axillary lymph node dissection) and vascular surgery.

2. Radiation Therapy: Radiation therapy, often used in cancer treatment, can damage or scar the lymphatic vessels and nodes, impairing their function and causing lymphedema in the irradiated area.

3. Cancer: In some cases, cancer itself can block or damage the lymphatic system. Lymphedema can occur as a result of cancerous tumours pressing on lymphatic vessels or nodes.

4. Infection: Infections of the lymphatic system, such as lymphangitis or cellulitis, can disrupt lymphatic function and lead to lymphedema. These infections may result from bacteria entering the lymphatic system through a wound or injury.

5. Inflammatory Conditions: Certain inflammatory conditions, such as rheumatoid arthritis, can cause inflammation and scarring of the lymphatic vessels, leading to lymphedema.

6. Trauma or Injury: Physical trauma, such as severe burns, severe contusions, or deep cuts, can damage lymphatic vessels or nodes, interfering with lymphatic drainage and causing localised lymphedema.

7. Congenital Conditions: Primary lymphedema is a rare congenital condition in which individuals are born with abnormalities in their lymphatic system. It may become evident in infancy, adolescence, or later in life.

8. Filariasis: In some parts of the world, filariasis is a parasitic infection that can harm the lymphatic system and cause swelling.

9. Obesity: Severe obesity can exert pressure on the lymphatic vessels, impairing their function and causing lymphedema, particularly in the lower limbs.

10. Venous Insufficiency: Chronic venous insufficiency, which is a condition where veins in the legs have difficulty returning blood to the heart, can lead to fluid accumulation and contribute to lymphedema in some cases.

It's important to note that lymphedema can develop immediately after surgery or radiation therapy, or it may appear months or even years later. While primary lymphedema is often present from birth or develops during childhood, secondary lymphedema is typically acquired later in life due to injury, surgery, or medical conditions.

Risk Factors for Lymphedema

can occur without any specific risk factors; certain factors may increase the risk of developing lymphedema. These risk factors include:

1. Cancer Treatment:

Lymphedema is commonly associated with cancer treatment, particularly when lymph nodes are removed or damaged during surgery or radiation therapy. For example, breast cancer treatment may involve axillary lymph node dissection, which increases the risk of arm lymphedema.

2. Type of Cancer:

• Certain cancers, such as breast cancer, gynaecological cancers, melanoma, and head and neck cancers, have a higher risk of lymphedema due to their proximity to lymph nodes and lymphatic vessels.

3. Surgery:

• Any surgery that involves the removal of lymph nodes or damage to the lymphatic system can increase the risk of lymphedema. This includes lymph node removal for diagnostic purposes or the treatment of conditions other than cancer.

4. Radiation Therapy:

• Radiation therapy can cause scarring and damage to lymphatic vessels and nodes, disrupting the normal flow of lymphatic fluid and increasing the risk of lymphedema in the treated area.

5. Infection:

• Repeated or severe infections of the lymphatic system, such as lymphangitis or cellulitis, can damage lymphatic vessels and nodes, potentially leading to lymphedema.

6. Obesity:

• Severe obesity can exert pressure on the lymphatic vessels and nodes, impairing their function and increasing the risk of lymphedema, particularly in the lower limbs.

7. Trauma or injury:

• Physical trauma, such as severe burns, severe contusions, or deep cuts, can damage lymphatic vessels or nodes, interfering with lymphatic drainage and increasing the risk of localised lymphedema.

8. Genetic Predisposition:

• Some individuals may have a genetic predisposition to developing lymphedema, even without an obvious trigger. This is more common in primary lymphedema cases, which are present from birth or develop later in life.

9. Filariasis:

• In some parts of the world, lymphedema can be caused by a parasitic infection called filariasis. The parasites block lymphatic vessels and nodes, leading to lymphedema.

10. Venous Insufficiency:

• Chronic venous insufficiency, a condition where veins in the legs have difficulty returning blood to the heart, can lead to fluid accumulation and contribute to lymphedema in some cases.

It's important to note that not everyone with these risk factors will develop lymphedema. Lymphedema risk can be reduced or managed through various measures, including early diagnosis and appropriate management of underlying conditions such as cancer, infection, or venous insufficiency. For individuals at higher risk due to cancer treatment or surgery, preventive measures and early intervention are essential to minimise the risk of lymphedema and manage it effectively if it does develop.

Stages and symptoms of lymphedema

Lymphedema is often categorised into stages based on the severity and progression of the condition. The staging systems can vary slightly, but here is a commonly used four-stage classification along with their peculiar symptoms:

Stage 0: Subclinical or Latent Lymphedema

• In this stage, there may be no visible swelling or obvious symptoms.

However, the lymphatic system is compromised or damaged.

• Peculiar Symptoms: Individuals may experience a feeling of heaviness, tightness, or discomfort in the affected area, even though there is no visible swelling. This stage can be challenging to diagnose based solely on symptoms.

Stage I: Mild Lymphedema

• In Stage I, there is mild, reversible lymphedema with swelling that typically reduces with limb elevation (elevation-dependent swelling).

• The swelling may be subtle and pitting, which means that when pressed, the skin retains an indentation that disappears when pressure is released.

• Peculiar Symptoms: The affected limb may feel full or slightly swollen, but the swelling usually decreases with rest and elevation. Some individuals may experience a sensation of tightness or discomfort.

Stage II: Moderate Lymphedema

• In this stage, lymphedema is moderate, and the swelling is persistent, even with limb elevation (non-elevation-dependent swelling).

• The skin may become more fibrotic and less elastic, and there may be areas of increased thickness or nodularity within the swelling.

• Peculiar Symptoms: The affected limb remains swollen and may feel heavy or achy. Skin changes, such as thickening or hardening, may become more noticeable.

Stage III: Severe Lymphedema

• Stage III is the most advanced stage of lymphedema, characterised by significant and often non-reducible swelling.

• The skin in the affected area may become thickened, fibrotic, and prone to infections.

• The limb may appear deformed, with pronounced fatty deposits and irregular contours.

• Peculiar Symptoms: Severe swelling, pronounced skin

changes, and potential complications such as recurrent infections are common. Pain, discomfort, and reduced mobility are also more likely in this stage.

It's important to note that not all individuals with lymphedema progress through all these stages, and the severity and progression can vary widely among affected individuals. Early diagnosis and intervention are crucial for managing lymphedema effectively and preventing its progression to more advanced stages.

Diagnosis of Lymphedema

The diagnosis of lymphedema typically involves a combination of clinical evaluation, medical history assessment, and, in some cases, imaging studies. The following are the key steps involved in diagnosing lymphedema:

1. Medical History and Symptom Assessment:

• Your healthcare provider will begin by taking a detailed medical history, including any history of cancer treatment, surgeries, injuries, infections, or other events that may have affected your lymphatic system.

• They will ask about your symptoms, including when they started, how they have progressed, and any factors that exacerbate or alleviate them.

• Information about any family history of lymphedema or related conditions may also be important.

2. Physical Examination:

• A physical examination is a crucial part of the diagnosis. Your healthcare provider will carefully examine the affected area(s) to assess the extent of swelling, skin changes, and any areas of discomfort or tenderness.

• They will compare the affected limb or area to the unaffected side to identify differences in size, texture, or temperature.

• During the examination, they may perform a stemmer sign test, gently pinching the skin at the base of the second toe or finger to assess for the presence of pitting oedema (an indentation that remains when pressure is applied).

3. Lymphatic Function Assessment:

• The healthcare provider may evaluate the function of your lymphatic system by measuring the rate of lymph flow or assessing lymphatic drainage patterns. This can help confirm the presence and extent of lymphedema.

4. Imaging Studies (Optional):

• In some cases, imaging studies may be used to help visualise the lymphatic system and confirm the diagnosis. These may include lymphoscintigraphy, magnetic resonance imaging (MRI), or lymphangiography. These tests can provide information about lymphatic flow, blockages, or structural abnormalities.

5. Exclusion of Other Conditions:

• Lymphedema may mimic other conditions, such as venous insufficiency or lipedema. To confirm a lymphedema diagnosis, your healthcare provider will need to rule out other possibilities through a physical examination and, if necessary, additional tests.

6. Specialist consultation:

• If lymphedema is suspected, you may be referred to a specialist experienced in the diagnosis and management of lymphedema, such as a lymphedema therapist, vascular specialist, or lymphedema clinic.

7. Measurement and documentation:

• Accurate measurement of limb circumference and regular documentation of changes in swelling are essential for monitoring lymphedema progression and response to treatment.

Key Differences Between Lymphedema And Lipedema

Lymphedema and lipedema are two distinct medical conditions that primarily affect the lymphatic system and can result in swelling of the limbs. While they share some similarities, they have different causes, underlying mechanisms, and treatment approaches. Here are the key differences between lymphedema and lipedema:

1. Causes:

• Lymphedema:

Lymphedema is caused by damage to or dysfunction of the lymphatic system. This damage can occur due to surgery, radiation therapy, infection, trauma, or congenital factors.

It is often secondary to another underlying condition or event that impairs lymphatic function, such as cancer treatment or surgery.

• Lipedema:

Lipedema is primarily a genetic condition, and its exact cause is not well understood. It is believed to be related to hormonal and genetic factors.

Unlike lymphedema, which is primarily associated with lymphatic system damage, lipedema is characterised by the abnormal accumulation of fat cells in the limbs.

2. Underlying Mechanisms:

- Lymphedema:

Lymphedema results from impaired lymphatic drainage. Damage to or removal of lymph nodes, lymphatic vessels, or lymphatic valves disrupts the normal flow of lymphatic fluid, leading to fluid accumulation in the tissues.

The swelling in lymphedema is primarily due to the accumulation of lymphatic fluid, and it can lead to fibrotic changes in the affected limb over time.

- Lipedema:

Lipedema is characterised by the abnormal growth and accumulation of fat cells, primarily in the legs and, in some cases, the arms. This fat buildup occurs despite a healthy diet and exercise.

The swelling in lipedema is predominantly due to the excessive growth of fat tissue, leading to enlarged limbs with a characteristic "column-like" appearance.

3. Affected Areas:

- Lymphedema:

Lymphedema can affect one or more limbs or body parts, depending on the extent of lymphatic system damage or dysfunction.

Swelling in lymphedema is typically localised to the area where lymphatic flow is impaired, and it often presents with a pitting appearance when pressed.

- Lipedema:

Lipedema primarily affects the lower limbs (legs and sometimes the thighs) and, to a lesser extent, the upper limbs (arms).

The swelling in lipedema is typically symmetrical, involving both limbs, and it does not involve the feet or hands. There is usually a clear demarcation at the ankles and wrists.

4. Onset and Triggers:

- Lymphedema:

Lymphedema can develop suddenly after surgical procedures or radiation therapy that affect lymph nodes and vessels. It can also occur years after treatment.

Infections, trauma, or other events that damage the lymphatic system can trigger lymphedema.

- Lipedema:

Lipedema typically begins during or after puberty, although it can also manifest during pregnancy or menopause.

Hormonal changes may play a role in the progression of lipedema.

5. Treatment:

- Lymphedema:

Lymphedema management often includes compression therapy, manual lymphatic drainage, exercise, and skin care. Surgical interventions may be considered in advanced cases.

Treatment focuses on reducing swelling, improving lymphatic flow, and preventing complications.

- Lipedema:

Lipedema management may involve conservative measures, including compression garments and lifestyle modifications. In some cases, liposuction can be considered to remove excess fat.

Treatment aims to manage symptoms and improve the appearance of the limbs.

◆ ◆ ◆

CHAPTER 2:

The Lymphatic System

The lymphatic system is a vital part of the human circulatory system and plays several essential roles in maintaining the body's health and overall function. It is a complex network of tissues, vessels, lymph nodes, and organs dedicated to fluid balance, immune defence, and nutrient transport. Here's an overview of the lymphatic system in the human body:

1. Lymph Fluid:

• The lymphatic system starts with lymph fluid, which is a clear, colourless fluid similar to blood plasma but without red blood cells.

• Lymph is derived from interstitial fluid, which bathes the body's cells, providing nutrients and removing waste products.

• Lymph fluid contains immune cells, proteins, and waste products, and it plays a crucial role in immune function.

2. Lymphatic Vessels:

• Lymphatic vessels are a network of thin-walled tubes that transport lymph fluid throughout the body.

• These vessels have one-way valves that prevent the backward flow of lymph, ensuring that it moves in one direction towards the heart.

3. Lymph Nodes:

• Lymph nodes are small, bean-shaped structures scattered throughout the lymphatic system.

• They serve as filters that trap and remove foreign particles, such as bacteria and viruses, from the lymphatic fluid.

• Lymph nodes contain immune cells called lymphocytes, which play a crucial role in the body's defence against infections.

4. Lymphatic Organs:

• In addition to lymph nodes, the lymphatic system includes lymphatic organs like the spleen, thymus, and tonsils.

• The spleen filters blood and plays a role in removing damaged blood cells and storing platelets.

• The thymus is important for the development of T lymphocytes, a type of immune cell.

• Tonsils are collections of lymphatic tissue located at the back of the throat and play a role in protecting against respiratory and oral infections.

5. Bone Marrow:

• Bone marrow is a major part of the lymphatic system and is responsible for producing lymphocytes (white blood cells), including B cells and T cells, which are crucial for immune function.

6. Function of the Lymphatic System:

• Maintaining Fluid Balance: The lymphatic system helps maintain fluid balance in the body by returning excess tissue fluid (lymph) to the bloodstream. This prevents the accumulation of fluid and swelling in the tissues.

• Immune Defence: The lymphatic system plays a critical role in the body's immune defense. Lymph nodes and lymphocytes within them help identify and fight infections by recognising and attacking pathogens.

• Nutrient Transport: The lymphatic system also transports dietary fats and fat-soluble vitamins (A, D, E, and K) from the digestive system to the bloodstream.

7. Lymphatic Circulation:

• Lymphatic fluid circulates throughout the body, moving through lymphatic vessels and passing through lymph nodes for filtration before returning to the bloodstream via larger lymphatic ducts.

• There are two main lymphatic ducts: the right lymphatic duct, which drains lymph from the right upper body, and the thoracic duct, which drains lymph from the rest of the body.

In summary, the lymphatic system is a crucial component of the body's immune defence and plays a vital role in maintaining fluid balance and nutrient transport. It works in tandem with the cardiovascular system to support overall health and wellness.

How Diet Affects Lymphatic Function

Diet can play a significant role in supporting lymphatic function in the body. A healthy diet can help maintain the overall health of the lymphatic system by providing essential nutrients, reducing inflammation, and promoting proper fluid balance. Here are several ways in which diet can assist lymphatic function:

1. Hydration: Adequate hydration is essential for proper lymphatic function. When the body is well-hydrated, lymphatic fluid can flow more easily. Drinking enough water helps prevent dehydration and ensures that lymphatic vessels can efficiently transport lymph throughout the body.

2. Nutrient-rich foods: A diet rich in vitamins, minerals, and antioxidants supports immune function and helps keep the lymphatic system healthy. Include a variety of fruits, vegetables, whole grains, lean proteins, and healthy fats in your diet to provide essential nutrients.

3. Antioxidants: Antioxidant-rich foods, such as berries, leafy greens, and citrus fruits, help protect lymphatic tissues and cells from oxidative stress. This can aid in the proper function of lymphocytes, which are crucial for the immune system.

4. Omega-3 Fatty Acids: Foods rich in omega-3 fatty acids, such as fatty fish (salmon, mackerel, and sardines), flaxseeds, and walnuts, have anti-inflammatory properties. Reducing inflammation can help support the overall health of the lymphatic system.

5. Low-Sodium Diet: Excessive sodium intake can lead to water retention and swelling, which may strain the lymphatic system. Reducing salt intake can help maintain proper fluid balance and reduce the risk of lymphatic congestion.

6. Fibre: High-fibre foods, such as whole grains, legumes, and vegetables, support digestive health. A healthy

digestive system is essential for the absorption of nutrients and the removal of waste products, which can indirectly benefit the lymphatic system.

7. Adequate Protein: Protein is essential for the repair and maintenance of tissues, including lymphatic vessels. Incorporate lean protein sources like poultry, fish, beans, and tofu into your diet.

8. Avoid Excessive Sugar and Processed Foods: Excess sugar and processed foods can contribute to inflammation and may negatively impact the lymphatic system. Reducing the consumption of sugary and highly processed foods is advisable.

9. Herbal Teas: Certain herbal teas, such as dandelion tea or ginger tea, are believed to have diuretic properties that may help reduce water retention and support lymphatic function. However, it's essential to consult with a healthcare provider before using herbal remedies.

10. Proper Portion Control: Overeating and excessive weight gain can put added pressure on the lymphatic system. Maintaining a healthy weight through portion control and balanced eating can support lymphatic health.

◆ ◆ ◆

CHAPTER 3:

Diet Recommendation for Lipedema and Lymphedema

Managing both lipedema and lymphedema through a nutritional approach involves maintaining a balanced and anti-inflammatory diet to support overall health, reduce swelling, and alleviate symptoms. The following are general nutritional guidelines for managing lipedema and lymphedema:

1. Maintain a balanced diet.

• Consume a balanced diet that includes a variety of whole foods, such as fruits, vegetables, whole grains, lean proteins, and healthy fats.

• Aim to include a range of colours in your fruits and vegetables, as different phytonutrients may have anti-inflammatory and antioxidant properties.

2. Hydration:

• Stay adequately hydrated to support lymphatic function. Drink water throughout the day to help lymphatic fluid flow efficiently.

3. Anti-Inflammatory Foods:

• Incorporate foods that are known for their anti-inflammatory properties, including fatty fish (e.g., salmon, mackerel), walnuts, flaxseeds, turmeric, ginger, and green tea.

• Omega-3 fatty acids, found in fish and certain plant sources, may help reduce inflammation.

4. Limit Sodium Intake:

• Excess sodium can contribute to water retention and swelling. Reduce sodium intake by minimising processed and high-sodium foods.

• Cook meals at home using herbs and spices for flavour instead of salt.

5. Adequate Protein:

• Include lean protein sources like poultry, fish, tofu, legumes, and dairy products in your diet. Protein is essential for tissue repair and maintenance.

6. Fibre-Rich Foods:

• High-fibre foods, such as whole grains, vegetables, and legumes, support digestive health and may help with nutrient absorption and waste elimination.

7. Portion Control:

• Maintain a healthy weight through portion control and balanced eating. Avoid overeating, as excessive weight can strain the lymphatic system.

8. Compression Garments and Nutrition:

• For individuals with lymphedema, compression garments should be worn as prescribed by healthcare professionals. Nutrition can complement compression therapy but should not replace it.

9. Herbal Teas:

• Certain herbal teas, such as dandelion tea, are believed to have diuretic properties that may help reduce fluid retention. Consult with a healthcare provider before using herbal remedies.

10. Individualised Guidance:

• Seek guidance from a registered dietitian or nutritionist with experience in managing lymphedema and lipedema. They can provide personalised dietary recommendations tailored to your specific needs and medical history.

11. Mindful Eating:

• Practicing mindful eating can help you become more aware of hunger and fullness cues. This can prevent overeating and promote healthy eating habits.

12. Stress Management:

• Manage stress through relaxation techniques, as chronic stress can exacerbate inflammation. Techniques such as deep breathing, meditation, and yoga may be beneficial.

Dietary Recommendation

Dietary recommendations for individuals with lipedema and lymphedema focus on promoting a healthy lifestyle, reducing inflammation, and maintaining a balanced diet. While there isn't a specific diet that can cure these conditions, proper nutrition can play a supportive role in managing symptoms and improving overall well-being. Here are some dietary recommendations, along with examples and scientific bases:

1. Balanced Diet:

• Scientific Basis: A balanced diet provides essential nutrients and supports overall health, which can help manage symptoms and reduce inflammation associated with lipedema and lymphedema.

• Examples:

o Include a variety of fruits and vegetables to provide vitamins, minerals, and antioxidants.

o Incorporate lean protein sources like poultry, fish, tofu, and legumes for tissue repair and maintenance.

o Choose whole grains (e.g., brown rice, quinoa, and whole wheat) for fibre and sustained energy.

o Opt for healthy fats, such as those found in avocados, nuts, seeds, and olive oil.

2. Omega-3 Fatty Acids:

• Scientific Basis: Omega-3 fatty acids have anti-inflammatory properties that may help reduce inflammation associated with lymphedema and lipedema.

• Examples:

o Fatty fish like salmon, mackerel, and sardines are rich in omega-3s.

o Plant-based sources include flaxseeds, chia seeds, walnuts, and hemp seeds.

3. Hydration:

• Scientific Basis: Staying well-hydrated is essential for maintaining lymphatic fluid balance and supporting overall health.

• Examples:

o Aim to drink water throughout the day.

o Herbal teas and infused water with lemon or cucumber are hydrating options.

4. Anti-Inflammatory Foods:

• Scientific Basis: Inflammation can exacerbate symptoms. Anti-inflammatory foods can help reduce inflammation.

• Examples:

o Turmeric and ginger contain compounds with anti-inflammatory properties.

o Incorporate these spices into your cooking or enjoy them in teas and smoothies.

5. Low Sodium Intake:

• Scientific Basis: High sodium intake can contribute to water retention and swelling, which may worsen symptoms.

• Examples:

o Limit processed and high-sodium foods.

o Cook meals at home using herbs and spices for flavour instead of salt.

6. Portion Control:

• Scientific Basis: Maintaining a healthy weight through portion control can reduce the strain on the lymphatic system and minimise symptoms.

• Examples:

o Practice mindful eating by paying attention to hunger

and fullness cues.

o Avoid overeating and prioritise balanced meals.

7. High-Fibre Foods:

• Scientific Basis: Fibre-rich foods support digestive health and may help with nutrient absorption and waste elimination.

• Examples:

o Include whole grains, legumes, vegetables, and fruits in your diet.

8. Herbal Teas:

• Scientific Basis: Some herbal teas, such as dandelion tea, are believed to have diuretic properties that may help reduce fluid retention.

• Examples:

o Consult with a healthcare provider before using herbal remedies.

9. Individualised Guidance:

• Scientific Basis: Nutritional needs can vary among individuals. Consulting with a registered dietitian or nutritionist can provide personalised dietary recommendations tailored to specific needs and medical histories.

Meal Planning For Lymphedema And Lipedema

Take note: For lymphedema

Day 1:

Breakfast:

• Greek yoghurt parfait with berries, honey, and a sprinkle of flaxseeds

• whole-grain toast.

Lunch:

• Grilled chicken salad with mixed greens, cherry tomatoes, cucumbers, and a vinaigrette dressing

• Quinoa salad with roasted vegetables

Snack:

• Sliced cucumber and carrot sticks with hummus

Dinner:

• Baked salmon with a lemon-dill sauce

• Steamed broccoli.

• Brown rice.

Day 2:

Breakfast:

• Oatmeal with sliced bananas, chopped walnuts, and a drizzle of honey

Lunch:

• Lentil and vegetable soup

• whole-grain crackers.

Snack:

• Greek yoghurt with a handful of mixed berries

Dinner:

• Grilled shrimp skewers with a side of quinoa

• Sautéed spinach with garlic.

Day 3:

Breakfast:

• Spinach and mushroom omelette with a side of whole-grain toast

Lunch:

• Turkey and avocado wrap with a whole wheat tortilla

• Mixed greens salad with balsamic vinaigrette

Snack:

• Sliced apple with almond butter

Dinner:

• Baked chicken breast with roasted sweet potatoes

• Steamed green beans

Day 4:

Breakfast:

• Smoothie with kale, banana, frozen berries, Greek yoghurt, and a splash of almond milk

Lunch:

• Quinoa and black bean salad with diced tomatoes, corn, and cilantro

Snack:

• Celery sticks with peanut butter.

Dinner:

• Grilled tofu with a teriyaki glaze

• Stir-fried broccoli, bell peppers, and carrots

• Brown rice.

Day 5:

Breakfast:

• Whole-grain waffles topped with sliced strawberries and a dollop of Greek yoghurt

Lunch:

• Mixed greens salad with grilled chicken, cherry tomatoes, and a lemon-tahini dressing

Snack:

• Cottage cheese with pineapple chunks

Dinner:

• Baked cod with a mango salsa

• Quinoa with roasted Brussels sprouts

Day 6:

Breakfast:

• Scrambled eggs with diced bell peppers, onions, and spinach

• whole-grain English muffin.

Lunch:

• Caprese salad with mozzarella, tomatoes, and fresh basil

• whole-grain crackers.

Snack:

• Sliced cucumbers and cherry tomatoes with a tzatziki dip

Dinner:

• Stir-fried lean beef with broccoli, snap peas, and carrots in a ginger-soy sauce

• Brown rice.

Day 7:

Breakfast:

• Overnight oats made with rolled oats, almond milk, chia seeds, and mixed berries

Lunch:

• Spinach and feta-stuffed chicken breast

• Steamed asparagus.

Snack:

• A small handful of mixed nuts

Dinner:

• Grilled shrimp and vegetable skewers with a side of quinoa

• Roasted Brussels sprouts with olive oil and balsamic glaze

Above is a 7-day meal plan for individuals living with lymphedema. It requires a focus on a balanced diet that includes anti-inflammatory foods and supports overall health. The plan provides a variety of nutrient-rich options to help manage symptoms and promote well-being. Ensure you drink plenty of water throughout the day to stay well-hydrated. This meal plan provides a foundation for a balanced diet, but individual preferences and dietary restrictions should be taken into account when creating a personalised plan for managing lymphedema.

Take note: For lipedema

Day 1:

Breakfast:

• Scrambled eggs with spinach and cherry tomatoes

• whole-grain toast.

· A small serving of mixed berries

Lunch:

· Grilled chicken breast salad with mixed greens, cucumber, and a balsamic vinaigrette dressing

· Quinoa or brown rice on the side.

Snack:

· Greek yoghurt with honey and a sprinkle of almonds

Dinner:

· Baked salmon with lemon and dill

· Steamed broccoli.

· Mashed sweet potatoes

Day 2:

Breakfast:

· Oatmeal with sliced bananas and chopped walnuts

· A drizzle of honey.

Lunch:

· Lentil soup.

· whole-grain roll.

Snack:

· Sliced apples with peanut butter

Dinner:

· Grilled shrimp with a garlic and herb marinade

· Sautéed spinach with garlic and olive oil.

· Quinoa.

Day 3:

Breakfast:

• Whole-grain pancakes with fresh berries and Greek yoghurt

Lunch:

• Turkey and avocado wrap with a whole wheat tortilla

• Mixed green salad with a vinaigrette dressing.

Snack:

• Carrot and celery sticks with hummus

Dinner:

• Baked chicken breast with rosemary and thyme

• Steamed green beans

• Brown rice.

Day 4:

Breakfast:

• Smoothie with kale, banana, frozen berries, Greek yoghurt, and almond milk

Lunch:

• Quinoa salad with chickpeas, diced cucumber, red onion, and feta cheese

Snack:

• Cottage cheese with pineapple chunks

Dinner:

• Baked cod with a mango salsa

• Roasted Brussels sprouts with olive oil and balsamic glaze

• Quinoa.

Day 5:

Breakfast:

• Whole-grain waffles with fresh strawberries and a dollop of Greek yoghurt

Lunch:

• Mixed greens salad with grilled chicken, cherry tomatoes, and a lemon-tahini dressing

Snack:

• Sliced cucumber and cherry tomatoes with a tzatziki dip

Dinner:

• Stir-fried tofu with broccoli, snap peas, and carrots in a ginger-soy sauce

• Brown rice.

Day 6:

Breakfast:

• Scrambled eggs with diced bell peppers, onions, and spinach

• whole-grain English muffin.

Lunch:

• Caprese salad with mozzarella, tomatoes, and fresh basil

• whole-grain crackers.

Snack:

• A small handful of mixed nuts

Dinner:

• Grilled lean beef or portobello mushrooms with asparagus and roasted sweet potatoes

Day 7:

Breakfast:

• Overnight oats made with rolled oats, almond milk, chia seeds, and mixed berries

Lunch:

• Spinach and feta-stuffed chicken breast

• Steamed asparagus.

Snack:

• Sliced apples with almond butter

Dinner:

• Grilled shrimp and vegetable skewers with a side of quinoa

• Roasted Brussels sprouts with olive oil and balsamic glaze

Above is a 7-day meal plan for individuals living with lipedema. This plan requires a focus on supporting overall health, maintaining a balanced diet, and potentially managing weight. On this plan, also ensure you drink plenty of water throughout the day to stay well-hydrated. Kindly take cognizance of your individual preferences and dietary restrictions.

◆ ◆ ◆

CHAPTER 4:

Recipes and Preparation

Omega-3 Fatty Acids:

Grilled Salmon with Lemon-Dill Sauce

Grilled Salmon with Lemon-Dill Sauce

Ingredients:

4 salmon fillets (6–8 ounces each)

2 tablespoons of olive oil

Salt and black pepper to taste

For the Lemon-Dill Sauce:

1/2 cup plain Greek yogurt

Zest of 1 lemon

Juice of 1 lemon

2 tablespoons fresh dill, finely chopped

1 clove garlic, minced

Salt and black pepper to taste

Instructions:

1. Prepare the lemon-dill sauce:

• In a small mixing bowl, combine the Greek yogurt, lemon zest, lemon juice, fresh dill, minced garlic, salt, and black pepper.

• Whisk the ingredients together until well combined.

• Taste the sauce and adjust the seasoning as needed. You can add more lemon juice for extra zing or dill for a stronger herb flavor. Set the sauce aside.

2. Preheat the grill.

• Preheat your grill to medium-high heat. Make sure the grates are clean and lightly oiled to prevent the salmon from sticking.

3. Season the salmon:

• Brush both sides of the salmon fillets with olive oil.

• Season the fillets with salt and black pepper to taste. The olive oil will help the seasoning adhere to the salmon.

4. Grill the salmon:

• Place the salmon fillets on the preheated grill, skin-side down (if your salmon has skin).

• Grill for about 4-5 minutes on each side, or until the salmon flakes easily with a fork and has a slightly charred appearance. Cooking time may vary depending on the thickness of the fillets.

5. Remove from Grill:

• Carefully remove the grilled salmon fillets from the grill and transfer them to a serving platter.

6. Serve with lemon-dill sauce.

• Drizzle the prepared lemon-dill sauce over the grilled

salmon fillets or serve it on the side as a dipping sauce.

7. Garnish and enjoy:

• Garnish the dish with additional fresh dill or lemon slices for extra flavor and presentation.

• Serve your grilled salmon with lemon-dill sauce alongside your favorite side dishes, such as steamed vegetables, quinoa, or a green salad.

Nutritional information (per serving, without side dishes):

• Calories: approximately 300–350 calories

• Protein: 35–40 grams

• Fat: 15-20 grams

• Carbohydrates: 5-7 grams

• Fiber: 0–1 gram

• Sugars: 2-3 grams

• Sodium: 200-250 milligrams

This grilled salmon with lemon-dill sauce is a flavorful and nutritious dish that's rich in protein and healthy fats. The lemon-dill sauce adds a refreshing and tangy element to complement the salmon's natural flavors. Serve it as a part of a balanced meal to support your lymphatic and overall health.

Mackerel Tacos with Mango Salsa

Ingredients: For the Mackerel Tacos:

• 4 mackerel fillets (about 4-6 ounces each)

• 2 tablespoons of olive oil

• 1 teaspoon ground cumin

• 1 teaspoon chili powder

- Salt and black pepper to taste
- 8 small whole wheat or corn tortillas
- 1 cup shredded red cabbage
- 1 cup diced cucumber
- 1/2 cup plain Greek yogurt (for topping)

For the mango salsa:

- 1 ripe mango, peeled and diced
- 1/2 red onion, finely chopped
- 1 jalapeño pepper, seeded and minced (adjust to your desired level of heat)
- 1/4 cup fresh cilantro, chopped
- Juice of 1 lime
- Salt to taste

Instructions:

1. Prepare the mango salsa.

- In a medium bowl, combine the diced mango, chopped red onion, minced jalapeño pepper, chopped cilantro, and lime juice.
- Season the salsa with a pinch of salt and stir to combine.
- Refrigerate the salsa while you prepare the mackerel and other taco ingredients.

2. Season the Mackerel:

- Pat the mackerel fillets dry with paper towels.
- In a small bowl, mix the ground cumin, chili powder, salt, and black pepper.
- Rub the spice mixture evenly on both sides of the

mackerel fillets.

3. Grill the Mackerel:

• Preheat your grill to medium-high heat and lightly oil the grates.

• Place the seasoned mackerel fillets on the grill.

• Grill for approximately 3–4 minutes per side, or until the fish flakes easily with a fork and has grill marks. Cooking time may vary depending on the thickness of the fillets.

4. Warm the Tortillas:

• While the mackerel is grilling, warm the tortillas in a dry skillet over medium heat or on the grill for about 30 seconds on each side. Keep them warm with a clean kitchen towel.

5. Assemble the tacos:

• To assemble each taco, place a mackerel fillet on a warmed tortilla.

• Top with shredded red cabbage and diced cucumber.

• Spoon a generous portion of mango salsa over the top.

• Drizzle with a dollop of plain Greek yogurt.

6. Serve and enjoy:

• Serve the Mackerel Tacos with Mango Salsa immediately.

• Garnish with extra cilantro or lime wedges, if desired.

Nutritional Information (per serving, including 2 tacos):

• Calories: Approximately 400-450 calories

• Protein: 25–30 grams

• Fat: 15-20 grams

• Carbohydrates: 35–40 grams

- Fiber: 5–6 grams
- Sugars: 10–12 grams
- Sodium: 350-400 milligrams

Sardine and Avocado Salad

Ingredients:

- 2 cans of sardines in olive oil, drained
- 2 ripe avocados, diced
- 1/2 red onion, finely chopped
- 1/2 cup cherry tomatoes, halved
- 1/4 cup fresh cilantro, chopped
- 1/4 cup fresh parsley, chopped
- Juice of 1 lemon
- 2 tablespoons extra-virgin olive oil
- Salt and black pepper to taste
- Optional: red pepper flakes for a bit of heat.

Instructions:

1. Prepare the Sardines:

- Drain the sardines from the olive oil and transfer them to a mixing bowl.
- Using a fork, gently break up the sardines into smaller pieces. Remove any large bones if present.

2. Dice the avocado.

- Cut the ripe avocados in half, remove the pits, and carefully dice the flesh. Add the diced avocado to the bowl with the sardines.

3. Add vegetables and herbs.

• To the bowl, add the finely chopped red onion, halved cherry tomatoes, chopped cilantro, and chopped parsley.

4. Prepare the dressing:

• In a small bowl, whisk together the lemon juice, extra-virgin olive oil, salt, and black pepper. Adjust the seasoning to your taste.

• If you like a bit of heat, you can add red pepper flakes to the dressing for some spiciness.

5. Toss and Serve:

• Drizzle the dressing over the sardine and avocado mixture in the bowl.

• Gently toss all the ingredients together until well combined and evenly coated with the dressing.

6. Serve and enjoy:

• Divide the sardine and avocado salad into individual servings.

• Garnish with additional cilantro or parsley, if desired.

• Enjoy your delicious and nutritious salad!

Nutritional information (per serving, approximately 1/4 of the recipe):

• Calories: approximately 320–350 calories

• Protein: 20–22 grams

• Fat: 25-28 grams

• Carbohydrates: 12–15 grams

• Fiber: 7-9 grams

• Sugars: 2-3 grams

• Sodium: 300-350 milligrams

Flaxseed-crusted baked tilapia

Ingredients:

- 4 tilapia fillets (about 6–8 ounces each)
- 1/2 cup ground flaxseeds
- 1/4 cup grated Parmesan cheese
- 1 teaspoon dried thyme
- 1/2 teaspoon paprika
- Salt and black pepper to taste
- 2 eggs, beaten
- Olive oil or cooking spray for greasing

Instructions:

1. Preheat the oven.

- Preheat your oven to 375°F (190°C).

- Grease a baking sheet with a light coating of olive oil or cooking spray to prevent sticking.

2. Prepare the flaxseed coating:

- In a shallow dish, combine the ground flaxseeds, grated Parmesan cheese, dried thyme, paprika, salt, and black pepper. Mix well.

3. Beat the Eggs:

- In another shallow dish, beat the eggs until well combined.

4. Coat the Tilapia:

- Dip each tilapia fillet into the beaten eggs, ensuring it's coated evenly.

5. Coat with Flaxseed Mixture:

• After dipping in the eggs, transfer the tilapia fillet to the flaxseed mixture.

• Press the fillet into the flaxseed mixture to coat both sides generously.

6. Place on the baking sheet:

• Place the coated tilapia fillets on the prepared baking sheet.

7. Bake the tilapia:

• Bake in the preheated oven for approximately 12–15 minutes, or until the tilapia is cooked through and the flaxseed coating is golden brown and crispy. Cooking time may vary based on the thickness of the fillets.

8. Serve and enjoy:

• Remove the baked tilapia from the oven and let it rest for a minute.

• Serve the flaxseed-crusted baked tilapia hot, garnished with fresh herbs or a squeeze of lemon juice if desired.

Nutritional information (per serving, one tilapia fillet):

• Calories: Approximately 250-280 calories

• Protein: 30-35 grams

• Fat: 12–14 grams

• Carbohydrates: 6–8 grams

• Fiber: 4-5 grams

• Sugars: 0–1 gram

• Sodium: 300-350 milligrams

Chia Seed Pudding with Berries

Ingredients:

• 1/4 cup chia seeds

• 1 cup unsweetened almond milk (or any milk of your choice)

• 1 tablespoon pure maple syrup or honey (adjust to taste)

• 1/2 teaspoon pure vanilla extract

• 1/2 cup mixed berries (such as strawberries, blueberries, or raspberries)

• Optional toppings: sliced almonds, additional berries, or a drizzle of honey

Instructions:

1. Mix chia seeds and liquid:

• In a mixing bowl, combine the chia seeds and unsweetened almond milk (or your preferred milk).

• Stir well to ensure the chia seeds are evenly distributed in the liquid.

2. Add sweetener and flavor.

• Add the pure maple syrup or honey (adjust the amount to your desired sweetness) and pure vanilla extract to the chia seed mixture.

• Stir again to incorporate the sweetener and flavor into the mixture.

3. Refrigerate and stir.

• Cover the mixing bowl and refrigerate the chia seed mixture for at least 2 hours or overnight. During this time, the chia seeds will absorb the liquid and thicken, creating a pudding-like texture.

• After about 30 minutes, give the mixture a stir to prevent clumping. Make sure to stir again before serving.

4. Prepare the berries:

• Wash and slice the mixed berries if needed. You can use a combination of strawberries, blueberries, raspberries, or your favorite berries.

5. Assemble and Serve:

• Once the chia seed pudding has reached your desired consistency (it should be thick and pudding-like), divide it into serving dishes or jars.

• Top each serving with the prepared mixed berries and any optional toppings you prefer, such as sliced almonds or extra berries.

• Optionally, drizzle a touch of honey over the top for added sweetness.

6. Enjoy:

• Serve your chia seed pudding with berries as a nutritious and satisfying breakfast or snack.

Nutritional information (per serving, without optional toppings):

• Calories: approximately 180–200 calories

• Protein: 4-5 grams

• Fat: 9-10 grams

• Carbohydrates: 22–25 grams

• Fiber: 10–12 grams

• Sugars: 7-9 grams

• Sodium: 80-100 milligrams

Walnut-crusted chicken tenders

Ingredients: For the Walnut Coating:

- 1 cup walnuts, finely chopped

- 1/2 cup whole wheat breadcrumbs (or gluten-free breadcrumbs if preferred)

- 1/4 cup grated Parmesan cheese

- 1 teaspoon dried thyme

- 1 teaspoon garlic powder

- Salt and black pepper to taste

For the chicken:

- 1 pound of boneless, skinless chicken tenders (or chicken breasts cut into strips)

- 2 large eggs, beaten

- Olive oil or cooking spray for greasing

Instructions:

1. Preheat the oven.

- Preheat your oven to 375°F (190°C).

- Line a baking sheet with parchment paper or lightly grease it with olive oil or cooking spray to prevent sticking.

2. Prepare the walnut coating:

- In a shallow dish, combine the finely chopped walnuts, whole wheat breadcrumbs, grated Parmesan cheese, dried thyme, garlic powder, salt, and black pepper. Mix well.

3. Coat the chicken:

- Dip each chicken tender into the beaten eggs, ensuring it's coated evenly.

4. Coat with Walnut Mixture:

- After dipping in the eggs, transfer the chicken tender to the walnut coating mixture.

• Press the coating onto the chicken to adhere it evenly to both sides.

5. Place on the baking sheet:

• Place the coated chicken tenders on the prepared baking sheet, leaving a little space between each.

6. Bake the chicken.

• Bake in the preheated oven for approximately 20–25 minutes, or until the chicken is cooked through and the walnut coating is golden brown and crispy. Cooking time may vary based on the thickness of the chicken.

7. Serve and enjoy:

• Remove the walnut-crusted chicken tenders from the oven and let them cool slightly.

• Serve the chicken tenders hot as a delightful and nutritious meal or snack.

Nutritional Information (per serving, approximately 3–4 chicken tenders):

• Calories: Approximately 350-400 calories

• Protein: 30-35 grams

• Fat: 20–25 grams

• Carbohydrates: 10–12 grams

• Fiber: 3-4 grams

• Sugars: 2-3 grams

• Sodium: 350-400 milligrams

Hemp Seed and Spinach Smoothie

Ingredients:

• 1 cup of fresh spinach leaves

- 1 banana, peeled and sliced
- 1/2 cup plain Greek yogurt
- 1 tablespoon hemp seeds
- 1/2 cup unsweetened almond milk (or any milk of your choice)
- 1 tablespoon honey (optional; adjust to taste)
- Ice cubes (optional, for a colder smoothie)

Instructions:

1. Prepare the ingredients:

- Wash the fresh spinach leaves thoroughly and remove any tough stems.

- Slice the banana into smaller pieces for easier blending.

2. Combine Ingredients:

- In a blender, add the fresh spinach leaves, sliced banana, plain Greek yogurt, hemp seeds, and unsweetened almond milk.

- If you prefer a sweeter smoothie, you can add honey at this stage. Adjust the amount to your desired level of sweetness.

3. Blend until smooth.

- Cover the blender and blend all the ingredients until you achieve a smooth and creamy consistency. If desired, you can add a few ice cubes during blending for a colder smoothie.

4. Check the consistency:

- After blending, check the consistency of the smoothie. If it's too thick, you can add a bit more almond milk and blend again until you reach your preferred thickness.

5. Serve and enjoy:

• Pour the hemp seed and spinach smoothie into a glass or jar.

• Enjoy your nutritious and delicious smoothie immediately.

Nutritional information (per serving):

• Calories: Approximately 250-300 calories

• Protein: 10–12 grams

• Fat: 8-10 grams

• Carbohydrates: 35–40 grams

• Fiber: 5–6 grams

• Sugars: 18–20 grams

• Sodium: 100-150 milligrams

Miso-Ginger Salmon Bowl

Ingredients:

For the Miso-Ginger Marinade:

• 2 tablespoons of white miso paste

• 2 tablespoons of low-sodium soy sauce

• 1 tablespoon grated fresh ginger

• 1 clove garlic, minced

• 1 tablespoon honey or maple syrup (optional for sweetness)

• Juice of 1 lime

• 2 salmon fillets (6–8 ounces each)

For the bowl:

• 2 cups cooked quinoa or brown rice

- 2 cups mixed greens (e.g., spinach, kale, and arugula)
- 1 cup sliced cucumber
- 1 cup shredded carrots
- 1/2 avocado, sliced
- 1/4 cup edamame (steamed and shelled)
- 2 tablespoons of sesame seeds
- Sliced green onions for garnish (optional)

Instructions:

1. Prepare the Miso-Ginger Marinade:

- In a small bowl, whisk together the white miso paste, low-sodium soy sauce, grated fresh ginger, minced garlic, honey or maple syrup (if using), and lime juice.

- Taste the marinade and adjust the sweetness or saltiness to your preference.

2. Marinate the salmon:

- Place the salmon fillets in a shallow dish or a resealable plastic bag.

- Pour the miso-ginger marinade over the salmon, making sure it's well coated.

- Cover the dish or seal the bag and refrigerate for at least 30 minutes to allow the salmon to marinate. You can marinate longer for enhanced flavor.

3. Preheat the grill or oven.

- Preheat your grill to medium-high heat or preheat your oven to 375°F (190°C).

4. Grill or bake the salmon:

- If grilling, lightly oil the grates to prevent sticking. Place the marinated salmon fillets on the grill.

• Grill for about 4-5 minutes per side, or until the salmon flakes easily with a fork and has a slightly charred appearance. Cooking time may vary depending on the thickness of the fillets.

• If baking, place the marinated salmon on a baking sheet lined with parchment paper. Bake for approximately 15-20 minutes, or until the salmon is cooked through.

5. Assemble the bowl.

• In serving bowls, divide the cooked quinoa or brown rice evenly.

• Top with mixed greens, sliced cucumber, shredded carrots, avocado slices, and steamed edamame.

6. Add the salmon.

• Once the salmon is cooked, place a salmon fillet on top of each bowl.

7. Garnish and serve:

• Sprinkle sesame seeds over the bowls and garnish with sliced green onions if desired.

• Serve the Miso-Ginger Salmon Bowl with additional lime wedges if you like.

Nutritional information (per serving):

• Calories: Approximately 500-550 calories

• Protein: 35–40 grams

• Fat: 20–25 grams

• Carbohydrates: 45–50 grams

• Fiber: 8–10 grams

- Sugars: 7-9 grams
- Sodium: 600-700 milligrams

Sesame-crusted tofu stir-fry

Ingredients:

For the sesame-crusted tofu:

- 1 block (14–16 ounces) of extra-firm tofu, pressed and cubed
- 1/4 cup sesame seeds
- 2 tablespoons whole wheat flour (or gluten-free flour)
- 1/2 teaspoon garlic powder
- 1/2 teaspoon onion powder
- Salt and black pepper to taste
- 2 tablespoons of low-sodium soy sauce
- 2 tablespoons of sesame oil for pan-frying

For the stir-fry:

- 2 cups mixed vegetables (e.g., bell peppers, broccoli, snap peas, and carrots), sliced
- 1 tablespoon sesame oil
- 2 cloves garlic, minced
- 1 tablespoon grated fresh ginger
- 2 tablespoons low-sodium soy sauce (or more to taste)
- 1 tablespoon honey or maple syrup (optional, for sweetness)
- Cooked brown rice or quinoa (optional, for serving)

Instructions:

1. Prepare the sesame-crusted tofu.

• Begin by pressing the tofu to remove excess moisture. Wrap the tofu block in a clean kitchen towel and place a heavy object (like a cast-iron skillet or cans) on top. Let it press for about 15–20 minutes.

• Once pressed, cut the tofu into bite-sized cubes.

2. Prepare the coating.

• In a shallow dish, combine the sesame seeds, whole wheat flour, garlic powder, onion powder, salt, and black pepper. Mix well.

• In another shallow dish, pour the 2 tablespoons of low-sodium soy sauce.

3. Coat the tofu:

• Dip each tofu cube into the soy sauce, ensuring it's coated.

• Then, coat the tofu cube with the sesame seed mixture, pressing gently to adhere the coating to all sides.

4. Pan-fry the tofu:

• In a large skillet or wok, heat 2 tablespoons of sesame oil over medium-high heat.

• Place the coated tofu cubes in the hot oil and cook for about 3–4 minutes per side, or until the sesame crust is golden brown and crispy. You may need to do this in batches.

• Once cooked, transfer the sesame-crusted tofu to a plate lined with paper towels to remove excess oil.

5. Prepare the Stir-Fry:

• In the same skillet or wok, add 1 tablespoon of sesame oil.

• Add the minced garlic and grated ginger. Stir-fry for about 30 seconds until fragrant.

6. Add Vegetables and Sauce:

• Add the sliced mixed vegetables to the skillet.

• Drizzle 2 tablespoons of low-sodium soy sauce (adjust to taste) and honey or maple syrup (if using) over the vegetables.

• Stir-fry the vegetables for about 4-5 minutes or until they are tender-crisp.

7. Combine tofu and vegetables:

• Return the sesame-crusted tofu to the skillet and gently toss everything together. Cook for an additional 1-2 minutes to heat the tofu.

8. Serve:

• Serve the sesame-crusted tofu stir-fry over cooked brown rice or quinoa, if desired.

Nutritional information (per serving, without rice or quinoa):

• Calories: Approximately 400-450 calories

• Protein: 15–18 grams

• Fat: 25-28 grams

• Carbohydrates: 25–30 grams

• Fiber: 5-7 grams

• Sugars: 8–10 grams

• Sodium: 650-750 milligrams

Crispy Skin Trout with Walnut Pesto

Ingredients:

For the walnut pesto:

• 1 cup fresh basil leaves, packed

- 1/2 cup walnuts, toasted
- 1/4 cup grated Parmesan cheese
- 2 cloves of garlic
- Juice of 1 lemon
- 1/4 cup extra-virgin olive oil
- Salt and black pepper to taste

For the Crispy Skin Trout:

- 4 trout fillets with skin on (6–8 ounces each)
- Salt and black pepper to season
- 2 tablespoons of olive oil

Instructions:

1. Prepare the walnut pesto:

- In a food processor, combine the fresh basil leaves, toasted walnuts, grated Parmesan cheese, garlic, and lemon juice.
- Pulse until the mixture is finely chopped.

2. Add olive oil and season.

- While the food processor is running, slowly drizzle in the extra-virgin olive oil until the pesto reaches your desired consistency.
- Season the pesto with salt and black pepper to taste. Set aside.

3. Prepare the Trout Fillets:

- Pat the trout fillets dry with paper towels. This step is essential for achieving crispy skin.
- Season both sides of the trout fillets with salt and black pepper.

4. Pan-Fry the Trout:

• In a large skillet, heat 2 tablespoons of olive oil over medium-high heat.

• Place the trout fillets in the skillet, skin-side down. Press down gently with a spatula to ensure even contact with the pan.

• Cook for about 3–4 minutes on the skin side, or until the skin is golden and crispy.

• Flip the fillets and cook for an additional 2-3 minutes on the flesh side, or until the trout is cooked through and flakes easily.

5. Serve with walnut pesto.

• Remove the crispy-skinned trout fillets from the skillet and place them on serving plates.

• Spoon a generous amount of walnut pesto over each fillet.

6. Garnish and enjoy:

• Garnish with additional fresh basil leaves and lemon wedges, if desired.

• Serve the crispy skin trout with walnut pesto immediately.

Nutritional Information (per serving, one trout fillet with pesto):

• Calories: Approximately 350-400 calories

• Protein: 30-35 grams

• Fat: 25-30 grams

• Carbohydrates: 5-7 grams

• Fiber: 2-3 grams

- Sugars: 1-2 grams
- Sodium: 350-400 milligrams

Anti-Inflammatory Foods:

Turmeric and Ginger Roasted Carrots

Ingredients:

- 1 pound of fresh carrots, peeled and trimmed
- 2 tablespoons of olive oil
- 1 teaspoon ground turmeric
- 1 teaspoon grated fresh ginger
- 1/2 teaspoon ground cumin
- Salt and black pepper to taste
- Fresh cilantro leaves for garnish (optional)

Instructions:

1. Preheat the oven.

- Preheat your oven to 425°F (220°C).

- Line a baking sheet with parchment paper or lightly grease it with olive oil.

2. Prepare the carrots.

- Peel and trim the fresh carrots. If they are thick, you can halve them lengthwise for even roasting.

3. Create the Turmeric and Ginger Spice Mix:

- In a small bowl, combine the olive oil, ground turmeric, grated fresh ginger, ground cumin, salt, and black pepper. Mix well to create a paste.

4. Coat the carrots:

- Place the prepared carrots in a mixing bowl.

- Drizzle the turmeric and ginger spice mix over the carrots.

- Toss the carrots until they are evenly coated with the spice mixture.

5. Roast the carrots:

- Spread the coated carrots in a single layer on the prepared baking sheet.

- Roast in the preheated oven for about 20–25 minutes, or until the carrots are tender and slightly caramelized. You can check for doneness by piercing a carrot with a fork; it should be easily pierced.

6. Garnish and serve:

- Remove the roasted carrots from the oven and transfer them to a serving platter.

- Garnish with fresh cilantro leaves, if desired.

- Serve the turmeric and ginger-roasted carrots hot as a nutritious and flavorful side dish.

Nutritional information (per serving, approximately 1/4 of the recipe):

- Calories: Approximately 80-100 calories

- Protein: 1-2 grams

- Fat: 7-8 grams

- Carbohydrates: 7-9 grams

- Fiber: 2-3 grams

- Sugars: 3–4 grams

- Sodium: 150-200 milligrams

Golden Turmeric Milk (Turmeric Latte)

Ingredients:

• 1 cup unsweetened almond milk (or any milk of your choice)

• 1/2 teaspoon ground turmeric

• 1/4 teaspoon ground cinnamon

• 1/4 teaspoon ground ginger

• A pinch of black pepper helps with turmeric absorption.

• 1 teaspoon honey or maple syrup (adjust to taste)

• 1/2 teaspoon coconut oil (optional)

• A small piece of fresh ginger, grated (optional)

• A small piece of fresh turmeric, grated (optional)

• Ground cinnamon or turmeric for garnish (optional)

Instructions:

1. Heat the milk.

• In a small saucepan, heat the unsweetened almond milk over medium heat until it's hot but not boiling. Stir occasionally to prevent scalding.

2. Mix in spices:

• Add the ground turmeric, ground cinnamon, ground ginger, and a pinch of black pepper to the hot milk.

• If you're using fresh ginger and fresh turmeric, add them as well.

• Stir the mixture well to combine.

3. Simmer and Infuse:

• Reduce the heat to low and let the mixture simmer for about 5–7 minutes. This allows the flavors to infuse.

4. Sweeten to Taste:

• Stir in the honey or maple syrup to sweeten the golden milk. Adjust the sweetness to your preference.

5. Add coconut oil (optional):

• If desired, add 1/2 teaspoon of coconut oil to the golden milk. This can provide a creamy texture and additional health benefits.

6. Strain (Optional):

• If you used fresh ginger and turmeric, you can strain the golden milk to remove any grated bits before serving.

7. Serve and garnish:

• Pour the golden turmeric milk into a cup or mug.

• If you like, garnish with a sprinkle of ground cinnamon or turmeric on top.

8. Enjoy:

• Sip and enjoy your soothing and nutritious golden turmeric milk. It's perfect for relaxing evenings or as a warming drink any time of the day.

Nutritional information (per serving):

• Calories: Approximately 60–70 calories

• Protein: 1-2 grams

• Fat: 2-3 grams

• Carbohydrates: 10–12 grams

• Fiber: 1-2 grams

• Sugars: 7-9 grams

• Sodium: 150-200 milligrams

Ginger-Lemon Chicken Soup

Ingredients:

• 1 pound of boneless, skinless chicken breasts or thighs, cut into bite-sized pieces

• 1 tablespoon of olive oil

• 1 onion, chopped

• 2 carrots, peeled and sliced

• 2 celery stalks, chopped

• 2 cloves garlic, minced

• 1-inch piece of fresh ginger, grated

• 6 cups low-sodium chicken broth

• Juice of 2 lemons

• Zest of 1 lemon

• 1 teaspoon ground turmeric

• Salt and black pepper to taste

• Fresh cilantro or parsley leaves for garnish (optional)

Instructions:

1. Sauté the chicken.

• In a large soup pot or Dutch oven, heat the olive oil over medium-high heat.

• Add the chicken pieces and sauté until they are lightly browned on all sides. Remove the chicken from the pot and set it aside.

2. Sauté the aromatics:

• In the same pot, add the chopped onion, sliced carrots, and chopped celery. Sauté for about 5 minutes, or until the vegetables begin to soften.

• Add the minced garlic and grated ginger. Sauté for an additional 1-2 minutes until fragrant.

3. Add broth and simmer.

• Return the sautéed chicken to the pot.

• Pour in the low-sodium chicken broth, lemon juice, and lemon zest.

• Stir in the ground turmeric, salt, and black pepper.

• Bring the soup to a boil, then reduce the heat to low. Cover and simmer for about 20–25 minutes, or until the chicken is cooked through and the vegetables are tender.

4. Adjust Seasoning:

• Taste the soup and adjust the seasoning by adding more salt, black pepper, or lemon juice if desired.

5. Serve:

• Ladle the ginger-lemon chicken soup into bowls.

• Garnish with fresh cilantro or parsley leaves if you like.

• Serve the soup hot and enjoy its comforting and nutritious flavors.

Nutritional information (per serving):

• Calories: Approximately 150-200 calories

• Protein: 20–25 grams

• Fat: 4-6 grams

• Carbohydrates: 10–12 grams

• Fiber: 2-3 grams

• Sugars: 4-6 grams

• Sodium: 400-500 milligrams

Turmeric and chickpea curry

Ingredients:

- 1 tablespoon of olive oil
- 1 onion, finely chopped
- 2 cloves garlic, minced
- 1-inch piece of fresh ginger, grated
- 2 teaspoons ground turmeric
- 1 teaspoon ground cumin
- 1 teaspoon ground coriander
- 1/2 teaspoon ground cinnamon
- 1/4 teaspoon cayenne pepper (adjust to taste)
- 1 can (15 ounces) chickpeas, drained and rinsed
- 1 can (14 ounces) diced tomatoes
- 1 can (14 ounces) coconut milk (full-fat or light)
- 2 cups fresh or frozen spinach or kale
- Salt and black pepper to taste
- Fresh cilantro leaves for garnish (optional)
- Cooked brown rice or quinoa for serving (optional)

Instructions:

1. Sauté the aromatics:

- In a large skillet or saucepan, heat the olive oil over medium heat.

- Add the chopped onion and sauté for about 3–4 minutes, or until it becomes translucent.

2. Add garlic and ginger.

• Add the minced garlic and grated ginger to the skillet. Sauté for an additional 1-2 minutes until fragrant.

3. Spice It Up:

• Stir in the ground turmeric, ground cumin, ground coriander, ground cinnamon, and cayenne pepper (adjust to your preferred level of spiciness). Cook for about 1 minute to toast the spices and enhance their flavors.

4. Add chickpeas and tomatoes.

• Add the drained and rinsed chickpeas and diced tomatoes (with their juices) to the skillet. Stir to combine.

5. Simmer with coconut milk:

• Pour in the can of coconut milk and stir well to incorporate.

• Bring the mixture to a gentle simmer and let it cook for about 10–15 minutes, allowing the flavors to meld together.

6. Add Greens:

• If using fresh spinach or kale, add it to the curry and let it wilt down. If using frozen greens, stir them in until heated through.

7. Season and Serve:

• Season the curry with salt and black pepper to taste.

• If desired, serve the turmeric and chickpea curry over cooked brown rice or quinoa.

8. Garnish and enjoy:

• Garnish with fresh cilantro leaves if you like.

• Serve the curry hot and savor its delicious flavors.

Nutritional information (per serving, without rice or

quinoa):

- Calories: Approximately 250-300 calories
- Protein: 6–8 grams
- Fat: 15-18 grams
- Carbohydrates: 25–30 grams
- Fiber: 7-9 grams
- Sugars: 5-7 grams
- Sodium: 500-600 milligrams

Grilled Turmeric and Honey Glazed Chicken

Ingredients:

For the Marinade:

- 4 boneless, skinless chicken breasts
- 2 tablespoons of olive oil
- 2 teaspoons ground turmeric
- 1 teaspoon ground paprika
- 1 teaspoon ground cumin
- 1/2 teaspoon ground coriander
- 2 cloves garlic, minced
- 2 tablespoons of honey
- Juice of 1 lemon
- Salt and black pepper to taste

For the Glaze:

- 2 tablespoons of honey
- 1 tablespoon of olive oil
- 1 teaspoon ground turmeric

- 1 teaspoon lemon zest
- Salt and black pepper to taste

Instructions:

1. Prepare the marinade.

- In a mixing bowl, combine the olive oil, ground turmeric, ground paprika, ground cumin, ground coriander, minced garlic, honey, lemon juice, salt, and black pepper.
- Mix well to create the marinade.

2. Marinate the chicken.

- Place the chicken breasts in a large resealable plastic bag or a shallow dish.
- Pour the marinade over the chicken, ensuring it's evenly coated.
- Seal the bag or cover the dish, and refrigerate for at least 30 minutes to marinate. For best results, marinate for 2-4 hours or overnight if time allows.

3. Preheat the grill.

- Preheat your grill to medium-high heat and oil the grates to prevent sticking.

4. Grill the chicken:

- Remove the chicken from the marinade and let the excess marinade drip off.
- Place the chicken breasts on the preheated grill.
- Grill for about 6–8 minutes per side, or until the chicken is cooked through and has nice grill marks.
- While grilling, baste the chicken with any remaining marinade for added flavor.

5. Prepare the glaze:

• In a small saucepan, combine the honey, olive oil, ground turmeric, lemon zest, salt, and black pepper.

• Heat over low heat, stirring continuously, until the glaze is well combined and slightly warmed. Remove from heat.

6. Glaze the chicken:

• During the last few minutes of grilling, brush the honey and turmeric glaze over the chicken breasts.

• Continue to grill for an additional 1-2 minutes per side, allowing the glaze to caramelize and create a flavorful coating.

7. Rest and Serve:

• Remove the grilled chicken from the heat and let it rest for a few minutes before slicing.

• Serve the grilled turmeric and honey-glazed chicken with your favorite side dishes or a fresh salad.

Nutritional Information (per serving, one chicken breast):

• Calories: approximately 300–350 calories

• Protein: 30-35 grams

• Fat: 9–11 grams

• Carbohydrates: 20–25 grams

• Fiber: 1-2 grams

• Sugars: 18–20 grams

• Sodium: 300-350 milligrams

Ginger and Spinach Smoothie

Ingredients:

• 1 cup of fresh spinach leaves

- 1 ripe banana
- 1/2 cup Greek yogurt (or dairy-free yogurt for a dairy-free option)
- 1/2 cup unsweetened almond milk (or any milk of your choice)
- 1 tablespoon fresh ginger, peeled and grated
- 1 tablespoon honey or maple syrup (adjust to taste)
- 1/2 teaspoon ground turmeric (optional)
- Ice cubes (optional)
- Chia seeds or flaxseeds for garnish (optional)

Instructions:

1. Prepare the ingredients:

- Wash and rinse the fresh spinach leaves.
- Peel and grate the fresh ginger.
- Peel and slice the ripe banana.

2. Combine Ingredients:

- In a blender, add the fresh spinach leaves, sliced banana, Greek yogurt, almond milk, grated ginger, honey or maple syrup, and ground turmeric if using.
- If you like your smoothie colder, you can also add a few ice cubes at this stage.

3. Blend until smooth.

- Cover the blender and blend all the ingredients until smooth and creamy. You may need to stop and scrape down the sides of the blender as needed.

4. Taste and adjust:

- Taste the smoothie and adjust the sweetness or ginger

flavor by adding more honey, ginger, or other ingredients to your liking.

5. Serve and garnish:

• Pour the ginger and spinach smoothie into a glass.

• If desired, garnish with a sprinkle of chia seeds or flaxseeds for added nutrition and texture.

6. Enjoy:

• Serve the smoothie immediately as a nutritious and refreshing drink.

Nutritional information (per serving):

• Calories: Approximately 250-300 calories

• Protein: 10–12 grams

• Fat: 3-5 grams

• Carbohydrates: 50–60 grams

• Fiber: 6–8 grams

• Sugars: 30-35 grams

• Sodium: 100-150 milligrams

Turmeric and Garlic Shrimp Stir-Fry

Ingredients:

For the stir-fry sauce:

• 2 tablespoons low-sodium soy sauce (or tamari for a gluten-free option)

• 1 tablespoon honey or maple syrup

• 1 teaspoon ground turmeric

• 1 teaspoon grated fresh ginger

• 2 cloves garlic, minced

- Juice of 1 lemon
- 1/4 cup of water
- 1 teaspoon cornstarch (or arrowroot powder for a gluten-free option)

For the stir-fry:

- 1 pound of large shrimp, peeled and deveined
- 1 tablespoon of olive oil
- 2 cups of broccoli florets
- 1 red bell pepper, sliced
- 1 yellow bell pepper, sliced
- 1 cup snap peas or snow peas
- 2 cloves garlic, minced
- Cooked brown rice or cauliflower rice for serving (optional)
- Fresh cilantro leaves for garnish (optional)
- Sliced green onions for garnish (optional)
- Sesame seeds for garnish (optional)

Instructions:

1. Prepare the stir-fry sauce:

- In a small bowl, whisk together the low-sodium soy sauce, honey or maple syrup, ground turmeric, grated fresh ginger, minced garlic, lemon juice, water, and cornstarch. Ensure the cornstarch is completely dissolved. Set aside.

2. Cook the shrimp:

- Heat the olive oil in a large skillet or wok over medium-high heat.

• Add the shrimp to the hot skillet and cook for about 2-3 minutes per side, or until they turn pink and opaque. Remove the cooked shrimp from the skillet and set them aside.

3. Sauté the vegetables.

• In the same skillet, add the broccoli florets, sliced red and yellow bell peppers, snap peas or snow peas, and minced garlic.

• Stir-fry the vegetables for about 4-5 minutes, or until they are tender-crisp.

4. Combine shrimp and sauce.

• Return the cooked shrimp to the skillet with the sautéed vegetables.

5. Add the stir-fry sauce.

• Pour the prepared stir-fry sauce over the shrimp and vegetables in the skillet.

• Stir well to coat the shrimp and vegetables evenly with the sauce.

6. Thicken the sauce.

• Cook for an additional 2-3 minutes, allowing the sauce to thicken and glaze the ingredients.

7. Serve:

• Serve the turmeric and garlic shrimp stir-fry hot over cooked brown rice or cauliflower rice, if desired.

• Garnish with fresh cilantro leaves, sliced green onions, and sesame seeds for added flavor and texture.

Nutritional information (per serving, without rice):

• Calories: Approximately 200-250 calories

- Protein: 20–25 grams
- Fat: 5-7 grams
- Carbohydrates: 20–25 grams
- Fiber: 4-6 grams
- Sugars: 10–12 grams
- Sodium: 500-600 milligrams

Spiced Sweet Potato Wedges with Turmeric Dip

Ingredients:

For the sweet potato wedges:

- 2 large sweet potatoes, washed and cut into wedges
- 2 tablespoons of olive oil
- 1 teaspoon ground cumin
- 1/2 teaspoon ground paprika
- 1/2 teaspoon ground coriander
- 1/4 teaspoon ground cinnamon
- Salt and black pepper to taste

For the Turmeric Dip:

- 1/2 cup Greek yogurt (or dairy-free yogurt for a dairy-free option)
- 1/2 teaspoon ground turmeric
- 1/2 teaspoon grated fresh ginger
- 1 clove garlic, minced
- Juice of 1/2 lemon
- Salt and black pepper to taste

Instructions:

1. Preheat the oven.

• Preheat your oven to 425°F (220°C).

• Line a baking sheet with parchment paper or lightly grease it with olive oil.

2. Season the sweet potato wedges:

• In a large mixing bowl, combine the sweet potato wedges, olive oil, ground cumin, ground paprika, ground coriander, ground cinnamon, salt, and black pepper.

• Toss the sweet potato wedges until they are evenly coated with the spice mixture.

3. Arrange on a baking sheet:

• Spread the seasoned sweet potato wedges in a single layer on the prepared baking sheet.

4. Bake the sweet potato wedges.

• Place the baking sheet in the preheated oven and bake for about 25–30 minutes, or until the sweet potato wedges are tender and crispy, turning them halfway through for even cooking.

5. Prepare the turmeric dip:

• While the sweet potato wedges are baking, prepare the turmeric dip. In a small bowl, combine the Greek yogurt, ground turmeric, grated fresh ginger, minced garlic, lemon juice, salt, and black pepper.

• Mix well to create the turmeric dip.

6. Serve:

• Once the sweet potato wedges are done baking and crispy, remove them from the oven.

• Serve the spiced sweet potato wedges hot with the

turmeric dip on the side.

Nutritional information (per serving, approximately 1/4 of the recipe):

- Calories: Approximately 150-200 calories

- Protein: 2-3 grams

- Fat: 6–8 grams

- Carbohydrates: 20–25 grams

- Fiber: 3-4 grams

- Sugars: 5-7 grams

- Sodium: 150-200 milligrams

Turmeric and Cumin-Roasted Cauliflower

Ingredients:

- 1 head of cauliflower, cut into florets

- 2 tablespoons of olive oil

- 1 teaspoon ground turmeric

- 1 teaspoon ground cumin

- 1/2 teaspoon ground coriander

- Salt and black pepper to taste

- Fresh cilantro leaves for garnish (optional)

- Lemon wedges for serving (optional)

Instructions:

1. Preheat the oven.

- Preheat your oven to 425°F (220°C).

- Line a baking sheet with parchment paper or lightly grease it with olive oil.

2. Prepare the cauliflower.

• Cut the cauliflower head into bite-sized florets.

• Place the cauliflower florets in a large mixing bowl.

3. Season the cauliflower:

• In a small bowl, combine the olive oil, ground turmeric, ground cumin, ground coriander, salt, and black pepper.

• Drizzle the spice mixture over the cauliflower florets.

4. Toss and coat:

• Toss the cauliflower florets until they are evenly coated with the spice mixture.

5. Roast the cauliflower:

• Spread the seasoned cauliflower florets in a single layer on the prepared baking sheet.

• Roast in the preheated oven for about 25–30 minutes, or until the cauliflower is tender and the edges are crispy, stirring once or twice for even cooking.

6. Garnish and serve:

• Once the cauliflower is done roasting, remove it from the oven.

• If desired, garnish with fresh cilantro leaves and serve with lemon wedges on the side for added flavor.

Nutritional information (per serving, approximately 1/4 of the recipe):

• Calories: Approximately 60–80 calories

• Protein: 2-3 grams

• Fat: 4-6 grams

• Carbohydrates: 6–8 grams

- Fiber: 2-3 grams
- Sugars: 2-3 grams
- Sodium: 100-150 milligrams

Ginger-Turmeric Green Tea

Ingredients:

- 1 green tea bag (or 1 teaspoon of loose green tea leaves)
- 1-inch piece of fresh ginger, thinly sliced
- 1/2 teaspoon ground turmeric (or 1 teaspoon grated fresh turmeric root)
- 1 teaspoon honey (optional; adjust to taste)
- 1 lemon slice (optional)
- Boiling water

Instructions:

1. Prepare the tea:

- Place the green tea bag (or loose green tea leaves) in a teapot or your favorite tea mug.

2. Add ginger and turmeric.

- Add the thinly sliced fresh ginger and ground turmeric (or grated fresh turmeric root) to the teapot or mug.

3. Pour boiling water:

- Carefully pour boiling water into the teapot or mug, covering the tea bag and ingredients.

4. Steep the tea:

- Allow the tea to steep for 3-5 minutes, depending on your desired strength. You can adjust the steeping time to suit your taste.

5. Sweeten (Optional):

• If desired, add honey to sweeten the tea. Adjust the amount to your preference. Stir until the honey is dissolved.

6. Garnish (Optional):

• For an extra touch of flavor and freshness, add a lemon slice to the tea.

7. Serve and enjoy:

• Remove the tea bag or strain the loose tea leaves if needed.

• Serve the ginger-turmeric green tea hot and savor its soothing and invigorating flavors.

Nutritional information (per serving):

• Calories: Approximately 5–10 calories (without honey)

• Protein: Negligible

• Fat: Negligible

• Carbohydrates: 1-2 grams

• Fiber: less than 1 gram

• Sugars: 0–1 gram

• Sodium: Negligible

Low Sodium Intake:

Homemade Low-Sodium Vegetable Broth

Ingredients:

• 1 large onion, roughly chopped

• 2 carrots, roughly chopped

• 2 celery stalks, roughly chopped

- 1 leek, trimmed, and roughly chopped
- 3 cloves garlic, minced
- 1 bay leaf
- 1/2 teaspoon whole black peppercorns
- 1/2 teaspoon dried thyme
- 1/2 teaspoon dried rosemary
- 1/2 teaspoon dried parsley
- 8 cups of water (approximately)
- Salt to taste (optional)

Instructions:

1. Prep the vegetables:

- Wash, peel, and roughly chop the onion, carrots, celery, and leek.
- Mince the garlic cloves.

2. Sauté the vegetables.

- In a large soup pot or Dutch oven, heat a small amount of water or olive oil over medium heat.
- Add the chopped onion, carrots, celery, leeks, and minced garlic.
- Sauté the vegetables for about 5-7 minutes until they start to soften and become fragrant.

3. Add herbs and spices.

- Add the bay leaf, whole black peppercorns, dried thyme, dried rosemary, and dried parsley to the sautéed vegetables.
- Stir to combine, and let the herbs and spices toast for a minute or two.

4. Pour in water.

• Pour in enough water to cover the vegetables, usually around 8 cups.

• Stir everything together.

5. Simmer the broth:

• Bring the mixture to a boil over high heat.

• Once it's boiling, reduce the heat to low and let the broth simmer uncovered for about 30–40 minutes, allowing the flavors to meld together and the vegetables to become tender.

6. Strain the Broth:

• After simmering, remove the soup pot from the heat and let it cool slightly.

• Strain the broth through a fine-mesh sieve or cheesecloth into a large bowl or another pot. Press down on the vegetables to extract all the liquid.

• Discard the solid remains.

7. Season (Optional):

• Taste the vegetable broth and season with a small amount of salt if desired. Remember that it's a low-sodium recipe, so use salt sparingly or omit it altogether.

8. Store or use:

• Let the vegetable broth cool completely before transferring it to airtight containers.

• Store the broth in the refrigerator for up to 3–4 days, or freeze it in portions for longer storage.

Nutritional Information (per cup, approximate):

• Calories: 10–15 calories

- Protein: Negligible
- Fat: Negligible
- Carbohydrates: 2-3 grams
- Fiber: 0–1 gram
- Sugars: 1-2 grams
- Sodium: minimal, depending on added salt

Baked Herb and Lemon Chicken

Ingredients:

- 4 boneless, skinless chicken breasts
- 2 tablespoons of olive oil
- 2 cloves garlic, minced
- 1 lemon, zest, and juice
- 1 teaspoon dried thyme
- 1 teaspoon dried rosemary
- 1 teaspoon dried parsley
- Salt and black pepper to taste
- Lemon slices for garnish (optional)
- Fresh parsley leaves for garnish (optional)

Instructions:

1. Preheat the oven.

- Preheat your oven to 375°F (190°C).
- Grease a baking dish with a small amount of olive oil or cooking spray.

2. Prepare the herb and lemon marinade:

- In a small bowl, combine the olive oil, minced garlic,

lemon zest, lemon juice, dried thyme, dried rosemary, dried parsley, salt, and black pepper.

• Mix well to create the marinade.

3. Marinate the chicken.

• Place the chicken breasts in the greased baking dish.

• Pour the herb and lemon marinade over the chicken, ensuring they are evenly coated.

• You can use your hands or a spoon to make sure the chicken is well covered with the marinade.

4. Bake the chicken.

• Place the baking dish in the preheated oven.

• Bake for approximately 25–30 minutes, or until the chicken is cooked through and no longer pink in the center. The internal temperature should reach 165°F (74°C).

5. Rest and garnish:

• Remove the baked herb and lemon chicken from the oven and let it rest for a few minutes.

• Optionally, garnish with lemon slices and fresh parsley leaves for added freshness and presentation.

6. Serve and enjoy:

• Serve the baked herb and lemon chicken hot with your choice of side dishes, such as steamed vegetables, brown rice, or a fresh salad.

Nutritional Information (per serving, one chicken breast):

• Calories: Approximately 200-250 calories

• Protein: 25–30 grams

• Fat: 8-10 grams

- Carbohydrates: 5-7 grams
- Fiber: 1-2 grams
- Sugars: 1-2 grams
- Sodium: 150-200 milligrams

Low-Sodium Taco Salad with Avocado Dressing

Ingredients:

For the salad:

- 1 pound of lean ground turkey or chicken
- 1 tablespoon of olive oil
- 1 small onion, finely chopped
- 2 cloves garlic, minced
- 1 teaspoon ground cumin
- 1 teaspoon chili powder
- 1/2 teaspoon paprika
- 1/4 teaspoon cayenne pepper (adjust to taste)
- Salt and black pepper to taste
- 6 cups mixed salad greens (e.g., lettuce, spinach, and arugula)
- 1 cup cherry tomatoes, halved
- 1/2 cup black beans, drained and rinsed (low-sodium)
- 1/2 cup corn kernels (fresh, frozen, or canned, without added salt)
- 1/4 cup diced red onion
- 1/4 cup sliced black olives (low-sodium)
- 1/4 cup chopped fresh cilantro (optional)

For the avocado dressing:

- 1 ripe avocado, peeled and pitted
- 1/4 cup Greek yogurt (or dairy-free yogurt for a dairy-free option)
- Juice of 1 lime
- 2 tablespoons fresh cilantro leaves
- 1 clove garlic, minced
- 2-3 tablespoons of water (adjust for desired consistency)
- Salt and black pepper to taste

Instructions:

1. Cook the ground turkey:

- In a large skillet, heat the olive oil over medium-high heat.

- Add the finely chopped onion and minced garlic and sauté for 2-3 minutes until they become fragrant and translucent.

- Add the ground turkey (or chicken) to the skillet and cook until it's browned and fully cooked, breaking it into smaller pieces as it cooks.

- Stir in the ground cumin, chili powder, paprika, cayenne pepper, salt, and black pepper. Cook for an additional 2–3 minutes to infuse the flavors. Set aside.

2. Prepare the avocado dressing.

- In a blender or food processor, combine the ripe avocado, Greek yogurt, lime juice, fresh cilantro leaves, minced garlic, water, salt, and black pepper.

- Blend until the mixture is smooth and creamy. Adjust the water to achieve your desired dressing consistency.

3. Assemble the salad:

• In a large salad bowl, layer the mixed salad greens as the base.

• Top the greens with the cooked and seasoned ground turkey (or chicken).

• Add the cherry tomatoes, black beans, corn kernels, diced red onion, sliced black olives, and chopped fresh cilantro (if using).

4. Drizzle with Avocado Dressing:

• Drizzle the creamy avocado dressing over the taco salad.

5. Serve and enjoy:

• Toss the salad gently to coat the ingredients with the dressing.

• Serve the low-sodium taco salad immediately and enjoy your delicious and nutritious meal.

Nutritional information (per serving):

• Calories: Approximately 350-400 calories

• Protein: 25–30 grams

• Fat: 15-20 grams

• Carbohydrates: 30-35 grams

• Fiber: 8–10 grams

• Sugars: 6–8 grams

• Sodium: approximately 200–300 milligrams (may vary based on ingredient choices).

Herb-Roasted Low-Sodium Potatoes

Ingredients:

• 1.5 pounds (about 4 cups) of baby potatoes (red or gold),

washed and halved

- 2 tablespoons of olive oil
- 2 cloves garlic, minced
- 1 teaspoon dried rosemary
- 1 teaspoon dried thyme
- 1 teaspoon dried oregano
- Salt and black pepper to taste
- Fresh parsley leaves for garnish (optional)

Instructions:

1. Preheat the oven.

- Preheat your oven to 425°F (220°C).

- Line a baking sheet with parchment paper or lightly grease it with olive oil.

2. Prepare the potatoes:

- Wash and halve the baby potatoes, keeping them a uniform size for even cooking.

3. Make the herb seasoning:

- In a small bowl, combine the olive oil, minced garlic, dried rosemary, dried thyme, dried oregano, salt, and black pepper.

- Stir well to create the herb seasoning.

4. Coat the potatoes:

- Place the halved baby potatoes in a large mixing bowl.

- Pour the herb seasoning over the potatoes and toss until they are evenly coated.

5. Arrange on a baking sheet:

• Spread the seasoned potatoes in a single layer on the prepared baking sheet.

6. Roast the potatoes:

• Place the baking sheet in the preheated oven and roast for about 25–30 minutes, or until the potatoes are golden brown and tender, stirring them once or twice for even cooking.

7. Garnish (Optional):

• If desired, garnish the herb-roasted low-sodium potatoes with fresh parsley leaves for a burst of color and freshness.

8. Serve and enjoy:

• Serve the potatoes hot as a delightful side dish or snack.

Nutritional information (per serving, approximately 1/4 of the recipe):

• Calories: Approximately 120–150 calories

• Protein: 2-3 grams

• Fat: 5-7 grams

• Carbohydrates: 18–20 grams

• Fiber: 2-3 grams

• Sugars: 1-2 grams

• Sodium: minimal, depending on added salt

Low-Sodium Tomato and Basil Bruschetta

Ingredients:

• 4 ripe tomatoes, diced

• 1/4 cup fresh basil leaves, chopped

• 2 cloves garlic, minced

- 2 tablespoons extra-virgin olive oil

- 1 tablespoon balsamic vinegar (low-sodium)

- Salt and black pepper to taste (minimal salt or salt substitute)

- 1 French baguette or whole-grain baguette, sliced

- Olive oil cooking spray (optional)

Instructions:

1. Prepare the tomatoes and basil.

- Wash and dice the ripe tomatoes.

- Chop the fresh basil leaves.

2. Make the tomato-basil mixture:

- In a mixing bowl, combine the diced tomatoes, chopped basil, minced garlic, extra-virgin olive oil, and balsamic vinegar.

- Season the mixture with minimal salt or a salt substitute and black pepper.

- Toss everything together gently to combine.

- Let the mixture sit at room temperature for about 15 20 minutes to allow the flavors to meld.

3. Toast the baguette slices:

- Preheat your oven's broiler on low.

- Arrange the baguette slices on a baking sheet.

- If desired, lightly spray the slices with olive oil cooking spray to help with browning.

- Place the baking sheet under the broiler and toast the slices for about 1-2 minutes per side, or until they are golden brown and crispy.

4. Top with Tomato-Basil Mixture:

• Once the baguette slices are toasted, remove them from the oven.

• Spoon the prepared tomato and basil mixture generously onto each toasted slice.

5. Serve and enjoy:

• Serve the low-sodium tomato and basil bruschetta immediately as a delightful appetizer or snack.

Nutritional Information (per serving, approximately 2-3 bruschetta slices):

• Calories: Approximately 80-100 calories

• Protein: 2-3 grams

• Fat: 3-4 grams

• Carbohydrates: 12–15 grams

• Fiber: 1-2 grams

• Sugars: 2-3 grams

• Sodium: minimal, depending on added salt

Grilled Low-Sodium Turkey Burgers

Ingredients:

For the turkey burgers:

• 1 pound of lean ground turkey

• 1/4 cup finely chopped onion

• 1/4 cup finely chopped bell pepper (any color)

• 2 cloves garlic, minced

• 1/4 cup fresh parsley, chopped

• 1 teaspoon dried oregano

- 1/2 teaspoon ground black pepper
- 1/4 teaspoon salt (or a salt substitute)
- Olive oil cooking spray

For serving (optional):

- Whole-grain burger buns or lettuce leaves
- Sliced tomatoes
- Sliced onions
- Lettuce leaves
- Mustard or low-sodium ketchup

Instructions:

1. Prepare the Turkey Burger Mixture:

- In a mixing bowl, combine the ground turkey, finely chopped onion, finely chopped bell pepper, minced garlic, fresh parsley, dried oregano, ground black pepper, and a minimal amount of salt or a salt substitute.

- Gently mix the ingredients until well combined. Be careful not to overmix, as this can make the burgers tough.

2. Form the Burger Patties:

- Divide the turkey mixture into four equal portions.

- With clean hands, shape each portion into a burger patty, about 1/2 to 3/4 inch thick.

3. Preheat the grill.

- Preheat your grill to medium-high heat, around 375–400°F (190-200°C).

- If using a stovetop grill pan or skillet, heat it over medium-high heat and lightly grease it with olive oil cooking spray.

4. Grill the turkey burgers:

• Place the turkey burger patties on the preheated grill or grill pan.

• Grill for about 4-5 minutes per side, or until the burgers are cooked through and reach an internal temperature of 165°F (74°C). Make sure to flip them gently to avoid sticking or breaking.

5. Serve the turkey burgers:

• If desired, lightly toast whole-grain burger buns on the grill.

• Assemble your low-sodium turkey burgers by placing each patty on a bun or lettuce leaf.

• Add sliced tomatoes, onions, lettuce leaves, and your choice of condiments, such as mustard or low-sodium ketchup.

6. Serve and enjoy:

• Serve the Grilled Low-Sodium Turkey Burgers hot with your favorite burger fixings.

Nutritional Information (per turkey burger patty, without bun and condiments):

• Calories: Approximately 150–160 calories

• Protein: 20–22 grams

• Fat: 7-8 grams

• Carbohydrates: 4-5 grams

• Fiber: 1-2 grams

• Sugars: 1-2 grams

• Sodium: minimal, depending on added salt

Low-Sodium Ratatouille

Ingredients:

- 1 eggplant, diced
- 2 small zucchinis, diced
- 2 small yellow squash, diced
- 1 red bell pepper, diced
- 1 yellow bell pepper, diced
- 1 orange bell pepper, diced (optional for added color)
- 1 onion, diced
- 2 cloves garlic, minced
- 1 can (14 oz) low-sodium diced tomatoes
- 2 tablespoons tomato paste (no salt added)
- 2 tablespoons extra-virgin olive oil
- 1 teaspoon dried basil
- 1 teaspoon dried thyme
- 1 teaspoon dried oregano
- Salt substitute or minimal salt (to taste)
- Black pepper (to taste)
- Fresh basil leaves for garnish (optional)

Instructions:

1. Prepare the Vegetables:

- Dice the eggplant, zucchinis, yellow squash, red bell pepper, yellow bell pepper, orange bell pepper (if using), and onion into uniform-sized pieces.

2. Sauté the Onions and Garlic:

• In a large, oven-safe skillet or Dutch oven, heat the extra-virgin olive oil over medium heat.

• Add the diced onion and minced garlic, and sauté for about 3-4 minutes until they become translucent and fragrant.

3. Add the Bell Peppers:

• Add the diced red, yellow, and orange bell peppers (if using) to the skillet.

• Sauté for another 2-3 minutes until the peppers begin to soften.

4. Add the Remaining Vegetables:

• Add the diced eggplant, zucchinis, and yellow squash to the skillet.

• Continue to sauté for an additional 5 minutes, stirring occasionally.

5. Season and Add Tomatoes:

• Stir in the dried basil, dried thyme, dried oregano, and black pepper.

• Pour in the low-sodium diced tomatoes (with their juice) and the tomato paste.

• If using a salt substitute, add it at this point to taste.

• Stir everything together to combine.

6. Simmer the Ratatouille:

• Reduce the heat to low, cover the skillet, and let the ratatouille simmer for about 20-25 minutes, stirring occasionally, until the vegetables are tender.

7. Garnish and Serve:

• If desired, garnish the Low-Sodium Ratatouille with fresh

basil leaves before serving.

• Serve it as a side dish or as a main course with whole grains like quinoa or brown rice.

Nutritional Information (per serving, approximately 1 cup):

• Calories: Approximately 70-80 calories

• Protein: 2-3 grams

• Fat: 3-4 grams

• Carbohydrates: 12-15 grams

• Fiber: 4-5 grams

• Sugars: 6-8 grams

• Sodium: Minimal, depending on added salt

Lemon Herb Quinoa (Using Minimal Salt)

Ingredients:

• 1 cup quinoa

• 2 cups water

• Zest of 1 lemon

• Juice of 1 lemon

• 2 tablespoons extra-virgin olive oil

• 2 cloves garlic, minced

• 1/4 cup fresh parsley, chopped

• 1/4 cup fresh cilantro, chopped

• 1/4 cup fresh chives, chopped

• Salt substitute or minimal salt (to taste)

• Black pepper (to taste)

• Lemon wedges for garnish (optional)

Instructions:

1. Rinse and Prepare Quinoa:

• Rinse the quinoa under cold water in a fine-mesh strainer to remove any bitterness.

• In a medium saucepan, combine the rinsed quinoa and 2 cups of water.

2. Cook Quinoa:

• Place the saucepan over high heat and bring it to a boil.

• Reduce the heat to low, cover the saucepan, and simmer for about 15-20 minutes, or until the quinoa is tender and the water is absorbed.

• Remove the saucepan from the heat and let it sit, covered, for 5 minutes.

3. Fluff Quinoa:

• After resting, use a fork to fluff the cooked quinoa to separate the grains.

4. Prepare Lemon Herb Dressing:

• In a small bowl, combine the lemon zest, lemon juice, extra-virgin olive oil, minced garlic, and a small amount of salt substitute or minimal salt.

• Season with black pepper to taste.

• Whisk the dressing until well combined.

5. Add Fresh Herbs:

• In a large mixing bowl, combine the cooked and fluffed quinoa with the chopped fresh parsley, cilantro, and chives.

6. Dress the Quinoa:

• Pour the lemon herb dressing over the quinoa and herbs.

• Toss everything together until the quinoa is evenly coated with the dressing.

7. Taste and Adjust Seasoning:

• Taste the Lemon Herb Quinoa and adjust the seasoning by adding more salt substitute or minimal salt and black pepper if needed.

8. Serve and Garnish:

• Serve the Lemon Herb Quinoa warm or at room temperature.

• If desired, garnish with lemon wedges for an extra burst of citrus flavor.

Nutritional Information (per serving, approximately 1 cup):

• Calories: Approximately 180-200 calories

• Protein: 5-6 grams

• Fat: 7-8 grams

• Carbohydrates: 27-30 grams

• Fiber: 3-4 grams

• Sugars: 0-1 grams

• Sodium: Minimal, depending on added salt

Low-Sodium Cucumber and Tomato Salad

Ingredients:

• 2 large cucumbers, thinly sliced

• 4 medium tomatoes, diced

- 1/4 red onion, thinly sliced (optional)
- 2 tablespoons extra-virgin olive oil
- 2 tablespoons white wine vinegar (low-sodium)
- 1 teaspoon dried oregano
- Salt substitute or minimal salt (to taste)
- Black pepper (to taste)
- Fresh basil leaves for garnish (optional)

Instructions:

1. Prepare the Vegetables:

- Wash and thinly slice the cucumbers.
- Dice the tomatoes into bite-sized pieces.
- Thinly slice the red onion if using.

2. Combine Cucumbers and Tomatoes:

- In a large mixing bowl, combine the sliced cucumbers, diced tomatoes, and thinly sliced red onion (if using).

3. Prepare the Dressing:

- In a small bowl, whisk together the extra-virgin olive oil, white wine vinegar, dried oregano, a minimal amount of salt substitute or minimal salt, and black pepper to taste.

4. Dress the Salad:

- Pour the dressing over the cucumber and tomato mixture.

5. Toss and Chill:

- Gently toss the salad to coat the vegetables evenly with the dressing.
- Cover the bowl and refrigerate for at least 30 minutes to allow the flavors to meld.

6. Garnish and Serve:

• Before serving, garnish the Low-Sodium Cucumber and Tomato Salad with fresh basil leaves if desired.

• Serve chilled as a refreshing side dish.

Nutritional Information (per serving, approximately 1 cup):

• Calories: Approximately 60-70 calories

• Protein: 1-2 grams

• Fat: 4-5 grams

• Carbohydrates: 6-8 grams

• Fiber: 2-3 grams

• Sugars: 3-4 grams

• Sodium: Minimal, depending on added salt

Roasted Low-Sodium Veggie Platter

Ingredients:

For the Veggie Platter:

• 2 cups broccoli florets

• 2 cups cauliflower florets

• 2 cups carrot sticks (about 2 medium carrots)

• 2 cups bell pepper strips (assorted colors)

• 2 cups zucchini rounds (about 2 medium zucchinis)

• 2 tablespoons extra-virgin olive oil

• Salt substitute or minimal salt (to taste)

• Black pepper (to taste)

• Fresh herbs for garnish (e.g., parsley, thyme, or rosemary) (optional)

For the Dipping Sauce (Optional):

- 1/2 cup plain Greek yogurt (low-fat or non-fat)
- 1 tablespoon lemon juice
- 1 teaspoon Dijon mustard
- 1 clove garlic, minced
- Salt substitute or minimal salt (to taste)
- Black pepper (to taste)

Instructions:

1. Preheat the Oven:

- Preheat your oven to 425°F (220°C).

2. Prepare the Vegetables:

- Wash and cut the broccoli and cauliflower into bite-sized florets.
- Peel and cut the carrots into sticks.
- Slice the bell peppers into strips.
- Slice the zucchinis into rounds.

3. Toss with Olive Oil and Seasonings:

- In a large mixing bowl, combine all the prepared vegetables.
- Drizzle the extra-virgin olive oil over the vegetables and toss to coat evenly.
- Season with a minimal amount of salt substitute or minimal salt and black pepper to taste. Toss again to distribute the seasonings.

4. Roast the Vegetables:

- Spread the seasoned vegetables in a single layer on a

baking sheet.

• Place the baking sheet in the preheated oven and roast for about 20-25 minutes, or until the vegetables are tender and lightly browned, stirring once halfway through.

5. Prepare the Dipping Sauce (Optional):

• In a small bowl, whisk together the plain Greek yogurt, lemon juice, Dijon mustard, minced garlic, and a minimal amount of salt substitute or minimal salt and black pepper to taste.

6. Garnish and Serve:

• Remove the roasted vegetables from the oven and transfer them to a serving platter.

• If desired, garnish with fresh herbs such as parsley, thyme, or rosemary.

• Serve the Roasted Low-Sodium Veggie Platter hot with the optional dipping sauce on the side.

Nutritional Information (per serving, approximately 1 cup of roasted veggies without dipping sauce):

• Calories: Approximately 60-80 calories

• Protein: 2-3 grams

• Fat: 3-4 grams

• Carbohydrates: 8-10 grams

• Fiber: 3-4 grams

• Sugars: 3-4 grams

• Sodium: Minimal, depending on added salt

High-Fiber Foods:

Whole Grain Berry Breakfast Parfait

Ingredients:

- 1 cup rolled oats (whole grain)

- 2 cups plain Greek yogurt (low-fat or non-fat)

- 2 cups mixed berries (e.g., strawberries, blueberries, raspberries)

- 2 tablespoons honey or maple syrup (optional for sweetness)

- 1/4 cup chopped nuts (e.g., almonds or walnuts)

- 1 teaspoon vanilla extract

- Fresh mint leaves for garnish (optional)

Instructions:

1. Prepare the Rolled Oats:

- In a dry skillet, toast the rolled oats over medium heat for about 5 minutes or until they become lightly golden and fragrant. Stir frequently to prevent burning.

- Remove from heat and let the toasted oats cool.

2. Prepare the Berries:

- Wash and chop the mixed berries into bite-sized pieces, if necessary.

3. Assemble the Parfaits:

- In serving glasses or bowls, start by layering about 1/4 cup of the toasted rolled oats at the bottom.

4. Add Yogurt Layer:

- Spoon approximately 1/4 cup of plain Greek yogurt on top of the oats in each glass.

5. Add Berries:

• Add a layer of mixed berries on top of the yogurt.

6. Drizzle with Sweetener (Optional):

• If you desire added sweetness, drizzle 1/2 to 1 tablespoon of honey or maple syrup over the berries in each glass.

7. Repeat Layers:

• Repeat the layering process by adding another 1/4 cup of toasted oats, followed by 1/4 cup of Greek yogurt, and another layer of mixed berries.

8. Garnish and Finish:

• Top each Whole Grain Berry Breakfast Parfait with a sprinkle of chopped nuts for added texture and flavor.

• Add a drop of vanilla extract to each parfait for extra aroma (optional).

• If desired, garnish with fresh mint leaves for a refreshing touch.

9. Serve:

• Serve the parfaits immediately as a nutritious and satisfying breakfast.

Nutritional Information (per serving, approximately 1 parfait):

• Calories: Approximately 350-400 calories

• Protein: 15-18 grams

• Fat: 10-12 grams

• Carbohydrates: 50-55 grams

• Fiber: 7-9 grams

• Sugars: 20-25 grams

• Sodium: Minimal

Chickpea and Vegetable Quinoa Bowl

Ingredients:

For the Quinoa Bowl:

• 1 cup quinoa

• 2 cups water or vegetable broth

• 1 can (15 ounces) chickpeas, drained and rinsed

• 2 cups mixed vegetables (e.g., bell peppers, zucchini, cherry tomatoes)

• 2 tablespoons olive oil

• 1 teaspoon ground cumin

• 1 teaspoon paprika

• 1/2 teaspoon garlic powder

• Salt substitute or minimal salt (to taste)

• Black pepper (to taste)

• Fresh parsley or cilantro leaves for garnish (optional)

For the Lemon-Tahini Dressing:

• 2 tablespoons tahini

• Juice of 1 lemon

• 2 tablespoons water

• 1 clove garlic, minced

• Salt substitute or minimal salt (to taste)

• Black pepper (to taste)

Instructions:

1. Prepare the Quinoa:

• Rinse the quinoa under cold water in a fine-mesh strainer

to remove any bitterness.

• In a medium saucepan, combine the rinsed quinoa and 2 cups of water or vegetable broth.

• Bring to a boil, then reduce the heat to low, cover, and simmer for about 15-20 minutes, or until the quinoa is cooked and the liquid is absorbed.

• Remove from heat, fluff with a fork, and let it sit, covered, for 5 minutes.

2. Roast the Chickpeas and Vegetables:

• Preheat your oven to 425°F (220°C).

• In a mixing bowl, combine the drained chickpeas, mixed vegetables, olive oil, ground cumin, paprika, garlic powder, a minimal amount of salt substitute or minimal salt, and black pepper to taste. Toss to coat evenly.

• Spread the seasoned chickpeas and vegetables in a single layer on a baking sheet.

• Roast in the preheated oven for about 20-25 minutes, or until the vegetables are tender and slightly caramelized.

3. Prepare the Lemon-Tahini Dressing:

• In a small bowl, whisk together the tahini, lemon juice, water, minced garlic, a minimal amount of salt substitute or minimal salt, and black pepper to taste. Adjust the consistency with more water if needed.

4. Assemble the Quinoa Bowl:

• Divide the cooked quinoa evenly among serving bowls.

• Top with the roasted chickpeas and vegetables.

5. Drizzle with Dressing:

• Drizzle the Lemon-Tahini Dressing over the quinoa,

chickpeas, and vegetables.

6. Garnish and Serve:

· Garnish the Chickpea and Vegetable Quinoa Bowl with fresh parsley or cilantro leaves if desired.

· Serve warm and enjoy!

Nutritional Information (per serving):

· Calories: Approximately 400-450 calories

· Protein: 10-12 grams

· Fat: 18-20 grams

· Carbohydrates: 55-60 grams

· Fiber: 9-11 grams

· Sugars: 5-6 grams

· Sodium: Minimal, depending on added salt

Lentil and Spinach Soup

Ingredients:

· 1 cup dried green or brown lentils, rinsed and drained

· 1 onion, chopped

· 2 cloves garlic, minced

· 2 carrots, diced

· 2 celery stalks, diced

· 1 can (14 ounces) diced tomatoes (low-sodium)

· 6 cups vegetable broth (low-sodium)

· 2 cups fresh spinach leaves, chopped

· 1 teaspoon ground cumin

· 1/2 teaspoon ground coriander

- 1/2 teaspoon smoked paprika
- Salt substitute or minimal salt (to taste)
- Black pepper (to taste)
- 1 tablespoon olive oil
- Fresh lemon juice (optional, for garnish)
- Fresh parsley leaves for garnish (optional)

Instructions:

1. Sauté the Vegetables:

- In a large pot or Dutch oven, heat the olive oil over medium heat.
- Add the chopped onion, minced garlic, diced carrots, and diced celery.
- Sauté for about 5 minutes, or until the vegetables begin to soften.

2. Add Spices:

- Stir in the ground cumin, ground coriander, and smoked paprika.
- Sauté for an additional 2 minutes to toast the spices.

3. Add Lentils and Broth:

- Add the rinsed lentils, diced tomatoes (with their juice), and vegetable broth to the pot.
- Season with a minimal amount of salt substitute or minimal salt and black pepper to taste.
- Bring the mixture to a boil.

4. Simmer:

- Reduce the heat to low, cover, and simmer for about 25-30 minutes, or until the lentils are tender.

5. Add Spinach:

• Stir in the chopped fresh spinach leaves and continue to simmer for an additional 2-3 minutes, or until the spinach wilts.

6. Adjust Seasoning:

• Taste the soup and adjust the seasoning as needed with salt substitute or minimal salt and black pepper.

• You can also add a squeeze of fresh lemon juice for a refreshing touch, if desired.

7. Garnish and Serve:

• Ladle the Lentil and Spinach Soup into bowls.

• Garnish with fresh parsley leaves if desired.

• Serve hot and enjoy!

Nutritional Information (per serving, approximately 1 1/2 cups):

• Calories: Approximately 250-280 calories

• Protein: 13-15 grams

• Fat: 4-5 grams

• Carbohydrates: 45-50 grams

• Fiber: 11-13 grams

• Sugars: 5-7 grams

• Sodium: Minimal, depending on added salt

Black Bean and Brown Rice Burrito Bowl

Ingredients:

For the Burrito Bowl:

• 1 cup brown rice (whole grain), cooked

- 1 can (15 ounces) black beans, drained and rinsed
- 1 cup corn kernels (fresh, frozen, or canned, low-sodium)
- 1 cup cherry tomatoes, halved
- 1 avocado, sliced
- 1/2 red onion, finely chopped
- 1 red bell pepper, diced
- 1/2 cup fresh cilantro leaves, chopped (optional)
- Salt substitute or minimal salt (to taste)
- Black pepper (to taste)

For the Lime-Cilantro Dressing:

- Juice of 2 limes
- 2 tablespoons olive oil
- 2 cloves garlic, minced
- 1/2 teaspoon ground cumin
- Salt substitute or minimal salt (to taste)
- Black pepper (to taste)

Instructions:

1. Cook the Brown Rice:

- Prepare brown rice according to package instructions. Once cooked, fluff it with a fork and let it cool.

2. Prepare the Lime-Cilantro Dressing:

- In a small bowl, whisk together the juice of 2 limes, olive oil, minced garlic, ground cumin, a minimal amount of salt substitute or minimal salt, and black pepper to taste. Set aside.

3. Assemble the Burrito Bowl:

• In individual serving bowls, start by layering cooked brown rice at the bottom.

4. Add Black Beans and Vegetables:

• Top the brown rice with black beans, corn kernels, halved cherry tomatoes, diced red bell pepper, sliced avocado, and finely chopped red onion.

5. Drizzle with Dressing:

• Drizzle the Lime-Cilantro Dressing over the assembled ingredients in each bowl.

6. Garnish:

• If desired, garnish each Black Bean and Brown Rice Burrito Bowl with fresh cilantro leaves for added flavor and color.

7. Season and Serve:

• Season the bowl with a minimal amount of salt substitute or minimal salt and black pepper to taste.

• Serve immediately and enjoy!

Nutritional Information (per serving):

• Calories: Approximately 400-450 calories

• Protein: 10-12 grams

• Fat: 15-18 grams

• Carbohydrates: 60-65 grams

• Fiber: 11-13 grams

• Sugars: 4-6 grams

• Sodium: Minimal, depending on added salt

Roasted Veggie and Lentil Salad

Ingredients:

For the Salad:

- 1 cup dried green or brown lentils, rinsed and drained
- 3 cups water or vegetable broth
- 2 cups mixed vegetables (e.g., bell peppers, zucchini, cherry tomatoes, red onion)
- 2 tablespoons olive oil
- 1 teaspoon dried thyme (or use fresh thyme leaves)
- Salt substitute or minimal salt (to taste)
- Black pepper (to taste)
- Fresh parsley or basil leaves for garnish (optional)

For the Balsamic Vinaigrette:

- 2 tablespoons balsamic vinegar
- 2 tablespoons olive oil
- 1 teaspoon Dijon mustard
- 1 clove garlic, minced
- Salt substitute or minimal salt (to taste)
- Black pepper (to taste)

Instructions:

1. Cook the Lentils:

- In a medium saucepan, combine the rinsed lentils and 3 cups of water or vegetable broth.
- Bring to a boil, then reduce the heat to low, cover, and simmer for about 20-25 minutes, or until the lentils are tender but not mushy.
- Drain any excess liquid and let the lentils cool.

2. Preheat the Oven:

• Preheat your oven to 425°F (220°C).

3. Prepare the Vegetables:

• Wash and chop the mixed vegetables into bite-sized pieces.

• Place them in a mixing bowl.

4. Toss with Olive Oil and Seasonings:

• Drizzle 2 tablespoons of olive oil over the chopped vegetables.

• Sprinkle dried thyme, a minimal amount of salt substitute or minimal salt, and black pepper to taste.

• Toss to coat the vegetables evenly.

5. Roast the Vegetables:

• Spread the seasoned vegetables in a single layer on a baking sheet.

• Roast in the preheated oven for about 20-25 minutes, or until the vegetables are tender and slightly caramelized, stirring once halfway through.

6. Prepare the Balsamic Vinaigrette:

• In a small bowl, whisk together balsamic vinegar, olive oil, Dijon mustard, minced garlic, a minimal amount of salt substitute or minimal salt, and black pepper to taste.

7. Assemble the Salad:

• In a large mixing bowl, combine the cooked lentils and roasted vegetables.

• Drizzle the Balsamic Vinaigrette over the salad.

8. Garnish:

• If desired, garnish the Roasted Veggie and Lentil Salad

with fresh parsley or basil leaves for added freshness.

9. Serve:

• Serve the salad warm or at room temperature as a hearty and nutritious meal.

Nutritional Information (per serving, approximately 1 1/2 cups):

• Calories: Approximately 350-400 calories

• Protein: 15-18 grams

• Fat: 15-18 grams

• Carbohydrates: 45-50 grams

• Fiber: 12-15 grams

• Sugars: 5-7 grams

• Sodium: Minimal, depending on added salt

Whole Grain Spaghetti with Tomato and Basil

Ingredients:

• 8 ounces whole grain spaghetti (or your preferred pasta)

• 2 cups fresh tomatoes, diced

• 2 cloves garlic, minced

• 1/4 cup fresh basil leaves, chopped

• 2 tablespoons extra-virgin olive oil

• Salt substitute or minimal salt (to taste)

• Black pepper (to taste)

• Red pepper flakes (optional, for a hint of spice)

• Grated Parmesan cheese (optional, for garnish)

• Fresh basil leaves for garnish (optional)

Instructions:

1. Cook the Pasta:

• Bring a large pot of water to a boil.

• Add a pinch of salt substitute or minimal salt if desired.

• Cook the whole grain spaghetti according to the package instructions until al dente.

• Drain and set aside, reserving a small amount of pasta cooking water.

2. Prepare the Tomato and Basil Sauce:

• While the pasta is cooking, heat 2 tablespoons of extra-virgin olive oil in a large skillet over medium heat.

• Add the minced garlic and sauté for about 1 minute until fragrant, being careful not to let it brown.

• Add the diced tomatoes to the skillet and sauté for about 2-3 minutes until they start to soften.

• Stir in the chopped fresh basil and season with salt substitute or minimal salt, black pepper, and red pepper flakes (if using).

• Continue to cook for another 2 minutes until the tomatoes break down slightly and release their juices.

3. Combine the Pasta and Sauce:

• Add the cooked and drained whole grain spaghetti to the skillet with the tomato and basil sauce.

• Toss the pasta with the sauce, using reserved pasta cooking water if needed to achieve your desired consistency.

4. Garnish and Serve:

• Garnish the Whole Grain Spaghetti with Tomato and Basil

with additional fresh basil leaves and grated Parmesan cheese, if desired.

• Serve hot and enjoy!

Nutritional Information (per serving, approximately 1 1/2 cups without cheese):

• Calories: Approximately 300-350 calories

• Protein: 8-10 grams

• Fat: 9-11 grams

• Carbohydrates: 48-52 grams

• Fiber: 6-8 grams

• Sugars: 3-5 grams

• Sodium: Minimal, depending on added salt

Quinoa Stuffed Bell Peppers

Ingredients:

For the Stuffed Bell Peppers:

• 4 large bell peppers (any color), tops removed, seeds and membranes removed

• 1 cup quinoa, rinsed and drained

• 2 cups vegetable broth (low-sodium)

• 1 can (15 ounces) black beans, drained and rinsed

• 1 cup corn kernels (fresh, frozen, or canned, low-sodium)

• 1 cup diced tomatoes (canned or fresh)

• 1/2 cup diced red onion

• 1 cup chopped spinach or kale (optional)

• 2 cloves garlic, minced

• 1 teaspoon ground cumin

- 1/2 teaspoon chili powder (adjust to taste)

- Salt substitute or minimal salt (to taste)

- Black pepper (to taste)

- 1 cup shredded low-fat cheese (optional, for topping)

Instructions:

1. Preheat the Oven:

- Preheat your oven to 375°F (190°C).

2. Cook the Quinoa:

- In a medium saucepan, combine the rinsed quinoa and vegetable broth.

- Bring to a boil, then reduce the heat to low, cover, and simmer for about 15-20 minutes, or until the quinoa is cooked and the liquid is absorbed.

- Fluff the quinoa with a fork and set aside to cool slightly.

3. Prepare the Bell Peppers:

- Cut the tops off the bell peppers and remove the seeds and membranes.

- If needed, trim the bottoms of the peppers slightly to help them stand upright in a baking dish.

4. Prepare the Filling:

- In a large mixing bowl, combine the cooked quinoa, black beans, corn, diced tomatoes, diced red onion, chopped spinach or kale (if using), minced garlic, ground cumin, chili powder, salt substitute or minimal salt, and black pepper.

- Mix well to combine all the ingredients.

5. Stuff the Bell Peppers:

• Carefully stuff each bell pepper with the quinoa and vegetable mixture, pressing down gently to pack the filling.

6. Bake:

• Place the stuffed bell peppers in a baking dish.

• If desired, top each pepper with a sprinkle of shredded low-fat cheese.

7. Cover and Bake:

• Cover the baking dish with aluminum foil.

• Bake in the preheated oven for about 30-35 minutes, or until the bell peppers are tender.

8. Remove from Oven and Serve:

• Carefully remove the stuffed bell peppers from the oven.

• Serve hot, garnished with fresh herbs if desired.

Nutritional Information (per stuffed bell pepper, without cheese):

• Calories: Approximately 300-350 calories

• Protein: 10-12 grams

• Fat: 2-4 grams

• Carbohydrates: 60-65 grams

• Fiber: 10-12 grams

• Sugars: 7-9 grams

• Sodium: Minimal, depending on added salt

Oat Bran and Blueberry Muffins

Ingredients:

• 1 cup oat bran

- 1 cup whole wheat flour
- 1/2 cup plain Greek yogurt (low-fat)
- 1/4 cup unsweetened applesauce
- 1/4 cup honey or maple syrup (for sweetness)
- 2 eggs
- 1 teaspoon baking powder
- 1/2 teaspoon baking soda
- 1/2 teaspoon ground cinnamon
- 1/4 teaspoon salt substitute or minimal salt
- 1 cup fresh or frozen blueberries
- 1/2 teaspoon vanilla extract
- Cooking spray or muffin liners

Instructions:

1. Preheat the Oven:

- Preheat your oven to 350°F (175°C).

- Prepare a muffin tin with cooking spray or line it with muffin liners.

2. Mix Dry Ingredients:

- In a large mixing bowl, combine oat bran, whole wheat flour, baking powder, baking soda, ground cinnamon, and a minimal amount of salt substitute or minimal salt.

- Mix the dry ingredients well.

3. Mix Wet Ingredients:

- In another bowl, whisk together plain Greek yogurt, unsweetened applesauce, honey or maple syrup, eggs, and vanilla extract until well combined.

4. Combine Wet and Dry Ingredients:

• Pour the wet ingredient mixture into the dry ingredients.

• Stir until just combined. Do not overmix; it's okay if there are a few lumps.

5. Add Blueberries:

• Gently fold in the fresh or frozen blueberries into the muffin batter.

6. Fill Muffin Cups:

• Spoon the muffin batter evenly into the prepared muffin cups, filling each about 2/3 full.

7. Bake:

• Place the muffin tin in the preheated oven and bake for approximately 18-20 minutes, or until a toothpick inserted into the center of a muffin comes out clean.

8. Cool and Serve:

• Allow the muffins to cool in the tin for a few minutes, then transfer them to a wire rack to cool completely.

Nutritional Information (per muffin, without added sweeteners):

• Calories: Approximately 120-140 calories

• Protein: 5-6 grams

• Fat: 2-3 grams

• Carbohydrates: 22-24 grams

• Fiber: 4-5 grams

• Sugars: 6-8 grams

• Sodium: Minimal, depending on added salt

Spinach and Chickpea Curry

Ingredients:

- 2 tablespoons olive oil
- 1 large onion, finely chopped
- 2 cloves garlic, minced
- 1-inch piece of fresh ginger, grated
- 1 teaspoon ground cumin
- 1 teaspoon ground coriander
- 1/2 teaspoon ground turmeric
- 1/2 teaspoon ground paprika
- 1/4 teaspoon cayenne pepper (adjust to taste)
- 1 can (15 ounces) chickpeas, drained and rinsed
- 1 can (14 ounces) diced tomatoes (low-sodium)
- 1 can (14 ounces) coconut milk (light or regular)
- 8 cups fresh spinach leaves, washed and chopped
- Salt substitute or minimal salt (to taste)
- Black pepper (to taste)
- Fresh cilantro leaves for garnish (optional)
- Cooked brown rice or whole grain naan for serving (optional)

Instructions:

1. Sauté Onions and Aromatics:

- Heat the olive oil in a large skillet or saucepan over medium heat.

- Add the finely chopped onion and sauté for about 5 minutes until it becomes translucent.

2. Add Garlic and Ginger:

• Stir in the minced garlic and grated ginger. Sauté for another 1-2 minutes until fragrant.

3. Spice it Up:

• Add ground cumin, ground coriander, ground turmeric, ground paprika, and cayenne pepper (if using).

• Stir the spices into the onion mixture and cook for about 1 minute until they become aromatic.

4. Add Chickpeas and Tomatoes:

• Add the drained and rinsed chickpeas to the skillet.

• Pour in the canned diced tomatoes (low-sodium) with their juice.

• Stir everything together and let it simmer for about 5 minutes.

5. Pour in Coconut Milk:

• Pour in the canned coconut milk (light or regular) and stir well to combine.

• Simmer the mixture for another 5-7 minutes until it thickens slightly.

6. Wilt the Spinach:

• Gradually add the chopped fresh spinach leaves to the skillet.

• Stir and cook until the spinach wilts down and combines with the curry, which should take about 2-3 minutes.

7. Season and Garnish:

• Season the curry with salt substitute or minimal salt and black pepper to taste.

• If desired, garnish with fresh cilantro leaves for added flavor.

8. Serve:

• Serve the Spinach and Chickpea Curry hot with cooked brown rice or whole grain naan, if you like.

Nutritional Information (per serving, curry only, without rice or naan):

• Calories: Approximately 250-300 calories

• Protein: 8-10 grams

• Fat: 16-18 grams

• Carbohydrates: 20-22 grams

• Fiber: 6-8 grams

• Sugars: 5-7 grams

• Sodium: Minimal, depending on added salt

Fruit and Nut Overnight Oats

Ingredients:

• 1/2 cup old-fashioned rolled oats

• 1 cup unsweetened almond milk (or your choice of milk)

• 1/4 cup Greek yogurt (low-fat)

• 1 tablespoon honey or maple syrup (for sweetness, optional)

• 1/4 teaspoon pure vanilla extract

• 1/4 cup mixed dried fruits (e.g., raisins, cranberries, chopped apricots)

• 2 tablespoons chopped nuts (e.g., almonds, walnuts, or your favorite)

• 1/2 cup fresh or frozen mixed berries (e.g., strawberries, blueberries, raspberries)

· Fresh mint leaves for garnish (optional)

Instructions:

1. Combine Oats and Liquid:

· In a glass jar or container, combine the old-fashioned rolled oats and unsweetened almond milk.

· Stir well to make sure the oats are fully immersed in the milk.

2. Add Greek Yogurt:

· Add the Greek yogurt to the oats and milk mixture.

· Stir to combine until the yogurt is well incorporated.

3. Sweeten and Flavor:

· If desired, add honey or maple syrup for sweetness and pure vanilla extract for flavor.

· Mix well to evenly distribute the sweetener and vanilla.

4. Add Dried Fruits and Nuts:

· Sprinkle the mixed dried fruits and chopped nuts over the oat mixture.

· Gently fold them in.

5. Incorporate Berries:

· Add the fresh or frozen mixed berries on top of the oat mixture.

· Do not stir the berries in at this point.

6. Cover and Refrigerate:

· Cover the glass jar or container with a lid or plastic wrap.

· Refrigerate the mixture for at least 4 hours or overnight. This allows the oats to absorb the liquid and flavors.

7. Serve and Garnish:

• When ready to eat, give the Fruit and Nut Overnight Oats a good stir to mix in the berries.

• Garnish with fresh mint leaves, if desired.

Nutritional Information (per serving):

• Calories: Approximately 300-350 calories

• Protein: 10-12 grams

• Fat: 8-10 grams

• Carbohydrates: 50-55 grams

• Fiber: 8-10 grams

• Sugars: 18-20 grams

• Sodium: Minimal, depending on ingredients used

◆ ◆ ◆

CHAPTER 5:

Exercise and Physical Activity

Exercise and physical activity can play a crucial role in managing both lymphedema and lipedema by promoting circulation, reducing swelling, improving muscle tone, and enhancing overall well-being. You should understand, as well, that exercise programs is also individualized and should be supervised by professionals, such as lymphedema therapists, physical therapists, or trainers experienced in working with lymphatic and lipedema conditions, especially for those with these two conditions.

The Role Of Exercise In Lymphatic Health

Exercise plays a significant role in maintaining and promoting lymphatic health. The lymphatic system relies on muscle contractions and physical movement to propel lymphatic fluid throughout the body. Exercise contributes to lymphatic health in the following ways:

1. Promotes Lymphatic Flow: Physical activity, particularly muscular contractions, aids in the movement of lymphatic fluid through the lymphatic vessels. When muscles contract and relax during exercise, they squeeze the

lymphatic vessels, helping to push lymph toward lymph nodes, where it can be filtered and cleansed.

2. Reduces Lymphatic Stagnation: Sedentary behavior can lead to lymphatic fluid stagnation, which may result in swelling and discomfort. Regular exercise helps prevent this stagnation by keeping the lymphatic fluid in motion.

3. Enhances Immune Function: Lymph nodes, which are critical components of the immune system, filter and trap harmful substances, such as bacteria and viruses, from the lymphatic fluid. Exercise can stimulate lymphatic flow through lymph nodes, potentially enhancing immune function.

4. Reduces Swelling and Edema: In conditions like lymphedema and lipedema, exercise, when done correctly and under the guidance of healthcare professionals, can help reduce swelling and edema by promoting lymphatic drainage.

5. Supports Weight Management: Maintaining a healthy weight through regular exercise can reduce the strain on the lymphatic system, as excess body weight can put added pressure on lymphatic vessels.

6. Improves Circulation: Exercise also supports overall blood circulation, which can indirectly benefit lymphatic health. Improved blood flow can enhance oxygen and nutrient delivery to cells, helping them function optimally.

7. Reduces Inflammation: Chronic inflammation can disrupt lymphatic function. Exercise has been shown to have anti-inflammatory effects, potentially aiding in the overall health of the lymphatic system.

8. Encourages Deep Breathing: Deep breathing exercises, often incorporated into physical activity like yoga and

Pilates, can create changes in pressure within the chest and abdomen, promoting lymphatic flow.

For Lymphedema:

1. Manual Lymphatic Drainage (MLD): MLD is a specialized massage technique performed by trained therapists to stimulate the lymphatic system and encourage the flow of lymphatic fluid. It can help reduce swelling and discomfort.

2. Compression Garments: Wear prescribed compression garments during exercise to support lymphatic drainage and reduce swelling. Ensure they fit correctly and provide adequate compression.

3. Low-Impact Aerobic Exercise: Engage in low-impact activities like walking, swimming, or cycling. These exercises promote circulation without placing excessive strain on the lymphatic system.

4. Range of Motion Exercises: Perform gentle range of motion exercises to prevent stiffness and maintain joint flexibility in the affected limb(s).

5. Strength Training: Light resistance training with proper technique can help improve muscle tone, which can assist in lymphatic fluid movement. Focus on both the upper and lower body.

6. Deep Breathing Exercises: Deep breathing and diaphragmatic breathing techniques can aid lymphatic flow by creating changes in pressure within the chest and abdomen.

7. Yoga: Yoga poses and gentle stretches can improve flexibility, circulation, and balance. Choose classes or poses that are suitable for your specific needs.

For Lipedema:

1. Low-Impact Cardio: Engage in low-impact cardiovascular activities like swimming, water aerobics, and cycling. These exercises can improve circulation without overexerting the lower limbs.

2. Resistance Training: Strength training can help increase muscle tone, which may improve the appearance of the limbs. Focus on both upper and lower body exercises.

3. Lymphatic Massage: Manual lymphatic drainage (MLD) or specialized massage techniques, performed by trained therapists, can help reduce pain and discomfort associated with lipedema.

4. Walking: Regular walking, especially brisk walking, can promote circulation and lymphatic flow. Start at your own pace and gradually increase intensity.

5. Leg Elevation: Spend time with your legs elevated above the heart level to reduce swelling. This can be incorporated into daily activities like reading or watching TV.

6. Stretching: Gentle stretching exercises can improve flexibility and reduce muscle tension, which may provide some relief from discomfort.

7. Deep Breathing: Deep breathing exercises can help with relaxation and potentially improve lymphatic flow.

General Exercise Tips:

· Due consultation as explained above.

· Wear properly fitted compression garments during exercise as prescribed.

• Start slowly and progress gradually. Listen to your body and avoid overexertion.

• Stay well-hydrated before, during, and after exercise.

• Pay attention to skin care and hygiene to prevent infections and irritation.

• Incorporate flexibility and balance exercises to maintain overall mobility.

◆ ◆ ◆

CONCLUSION

In conclusion, the book "Lymphedema and Lipedema Nutrition Guide" serves as a comprehensive resource that delves into the intricate relationship between diet and the management of these two unique medical conditions. Lymphedema and lipedema, though distinct in nature, share a common need for thoughtful and tailored nutritional strategies to enhance the overall well-being of individuals living with these conditions.

Throughout the pages of this book, we have explored the scientific basis behind various dietary approaches, such as incorporating omega-3 fatty acids to combat inflammation, embracing anti-inflammatory foods like turmeric and ginger, practicing low sodium intake to manage swelling, and prioritizing high-fiber foods to support digestive health. These dietary recommendations are not only rooted in scientific understanding but also take into account the specific needs and challenges faced by those with lymphedema and lipedema.

Furthermore, the book has offered practical insights into the development of meal plans tailored to these conditions, providing a foundation for balanced and nourishing diets that can contribute to symptom management and an improved quality of life. From breakfast to dinner, these meal plans are designed to inspire and empower individuals to make informed dietary choices that align with their unique health goals.

Beyond diet, the book has emphasized the importance of a holistic approach to managing lymphedema and lipedema, recognizing the integral role of exercise and physical activity in promoting circulation, reducing swelling, and enhancing lymphatic health. It has underscored the significance of seeking guidance from healthcare professionals who specialize in these conditions, ensuring that dietary and exercise plans are safe and individually tailored.

In the journey to manage lymphedema and lipedema, it is essential to remember that there is no one-size-fits-all solution. Each individual's experience is unique, and personalized care is paramount. By embracing the principles and recommendations outlined in this book, individuals can take proactive steps towards managing their conditions, improving their overall well-being, and enhancing their quality of life.

As we conclude this nutrition guide, we encourage readers to approach their health journey with a spirit of empowerment and resilience. By combining the knowledge within these pages with the guidance of healthcare professionals, individuals can embark on a path toward better nutrition, improved lymphatic health, and a brighter future in the face of lymphedema and lipedema.

Made in the USA
Monee, IL
29 February 2024

e88cf0db-56bf-410c-af49-ef8dfe99259cR01